Do No Harm

Do No Harm

A Personal Memoir

A. Stuart Hanson, MD

Wolfe Lake Press

Do No Harm
A Personal Memoir
All Rights Reserved.
Copyright © 2020 A. Stuart Hanson MD
v1.0

The opinions expressed in this manuscript are solely the opinions of the author and do not represent the opinions or thoughts of the publisher. The author has represented and warranted full ownership and/or legal right to publish all the materials in this book.

This book may not be reproduced, transmitted, or stored in whole or in part by any means, including graphic, electronic, or mechanical without the express written consent of the publisher except in the case of brief quotations embodied in critical articles and reviews.

Wolfe Lake Press

ISBN: 978-1-7923-2527-4

Cover Photo © 2020 A. Stuart Hanson MD. All Rights Reserved – Used With Permission.

PRINTED IN THE UNITED STATES OF AMERICA

To Art and Fran, my parents, who started this journey

To Gail, my wife, who enhances it daily by sharing her life with me

To Marta and Peter, our daughter and son, who continue to bring us joy

To Halen, Peter and Elise's son, who is our only grandchild

To Kelly, Marta's wife, who enhances our family

To Eileen, my sister, who shared our childhood

To Halen's mother Elise and husband Rob, who include us in their family,
and

To any future generations who might read these stories

Contents

Introduction *xi*

Youth
1 Fifteenth and Fifty-Third *5*
2 Lessons from Lying *11*
3 Ball Sports *13*
4 Who Do You Want to Be? *21*
5 Immigrant Farms *29*
6 Canoes, Camps, and Cabins *47*
7 Championship Seasons *59*

Becoming an Adult
8 Athletics and Academics *73*
9 Summer of 1961 *81*
10 Behind the Iron Curtain *89*

Family and Work
11 Finding Love *101*
12 The General *111*
13 Our Introduction to Asia *127*
14 War Zone *135*
15 Life on the Beach *141*
16 The Road Less Traveled *151*
17 Accidental Trafficking *157*
18 Teaching Sex in Sunday School *165*
19 Go by Land *171*

A Physician's Life
20 Pulmonary Medicine   *181*
21 My Practice Meets the Law   *187*
22 Stillwater Prison   *199*
23 Clearing the Air   *207*
24 An Unexpected Reunion   *221*

Closing Thoughts
25 The Final Chapter   *233*
26 Beliefs, Values, and My Lists   *239*

Acknowledgments

These memoirs would not have been written without the continuing encouragement of my family. Our daughter, Marta, is an East Asian public health historian and has motivated me to record some of my experiences. Peter, our son, is a sports medicine physician and encouraged recording the stories we tell at our family gatherings. My sister, Eileen Hanson-Kelly, has read each chapter as it was written and made both editorial comments and historical corrections. My brother-in-law, Robert Taylor, a published memoirist, has given me insight and encouragement along the way.

Park Nicollet and its predecessor organizations have been supportive especially of my interests in public health and public policy. Bud Green, Arnie Anderson, Norm Sterrie, Glen Nelson, and Roger Asplin were instrumental in giving me the space early in my career to get involved in health-care organizations outside of the organization that paid me.

The colleagues at Park Nicollet supported me when my activities were not popular inside and outside of our pulmonary practice. Dick Woellner, Will Corson, Tom Dunkel, Bill Schoenwetter, David Randall, and Mark Wedel were the colleagues who supported the initiatives in smoke-free workplaces. Later, Keith Harmon, Kevin Komadina, Salim Kathawala, Sue Ravenscraft, Azra Mouhiddin, Laural Wright, Nicki Myers, Lisa Bolin, Amy Cashman, and Mandy Anderson taught me how to be a caring physician and made my medical-practice life a joy.

I am indebted to the public health community in Minnesota who have shared opportunities to improve the health of populations. I want to especially thank Paul Blake and Paul Olfeldt for getting me started within organized medical societies. Jeanne Weigum, Judy Knapp, Tom Kottke, Dick Neimic, Roger Johnson, Pat McComes, Sandy Sandel, Jim Hart, and Richard Hurt greatly enhanced my understanding of tobacco control and public health and motivated me when failures arrived.

Jim Toscano, Paul Terry, Jinnet Fowles, Richard Bergenstal, Roger Mazzie, Ellie Strock, Mary Heinz, Mary Pappas, and Ruth Spellmon were instrumental in any success we had with the Park Nicollet Institute for Research and Education.

In 2015 I was introduced to Joe Kita who led a course on memoir writing aboard the *Crystal Serenity* cruise ship. His lectures and advice have been instrumental in understanding the memoirs genre and the process of publishing a book. I thank the editors at Minnesota Medicine and Geisel Medical School at Dartmouth for editing my drafts and their advice on using proper names.

Kitty Czarniecki has been a wonderful editor and advisor on shaping a collection of stories into what I hope is a readable book. Always diplomatic in her recommendations, she made my writing better. Dorie McClelland has taken my digital files and old photographs and somehow transformed them into an attractive book. Without Joe, Kitty, and Dorie this book would not have been possible.

My wife, Gail, an English teacher and PhD organization-communications educator, has given me constant support. Her input has been an essential resource. I thank her for her loving devotion to our lives together. Without her, most of these events and the resulting stories would not have happened.

Introduction

I began these writings at the request of my family. Many of the stories in this memoir have been told by me and other family members around dinner tables and other social gatherings. Mostly the chapters are written from memory, but I do have access to family letters and travel journals. I found them somewhat helpful, but at times a distraction. Some of my letters from behind the Iron Curtain are not fully truthful due to the circumstances of movement in a hostile region of the world.

Others who experienced some of the events depicted here may have different memories or interpretations. The process of retrieving the past through one's memory and notes can be subjective, but even documents made at the time of an event by their nature are not necessarily totally objective. I have tried to be as true as possible to the actual events. Where dialogue is used, I have tried to be as specific as I remember it when no actual recording was available.

Excerpts from four of the chapters have been previously published. "Clearing the Air," "Stillwater Prison," and "My Practice Meets the Law" were published in *Minnesota Medicine*. "An Unexpected Reunion" was published in the *Geisel School of Medicine at Dartmouth, Alumni News*. They have been modified and updated for this publication.

The chapters are laid out as they seemed to fit best in a book. It is not meant to be an autobiography, but a selective memoir of events and thoughts. I have tried to make each chapter self contained, so it could be read as an independent essay, and I have tried not to repeat myself. I expect some readers will find I have not meet those goals, for which I apologize. I have grouped chapters into sections that are self explanatory in hopes they will clue readers to my thinking.

Recounting past experiences has been an enjoyable experience. Having the luxury of time has given me the opportunity to recall and reflect on what happened and what didn't happen. That has been the most rewarding result for me of this endeavor. These are my memories and I have tried to put them in a readable form. I take responsibility for what I have written and apologize to the reader for any inaccuracies or misinterpretations that I may have made.

Do No Harm

Youth

CHAPTER ONE

Fifteenth and Fifty-Third

I grew up in south Minneapolis, "Fifteenth and Fifty-Third." We lived on Fifteenth Avenue three houses from Fifty-Third Street. Because each house was located on a forty-foot-wide lot, the streets became our play fields as we dodged the occasional passing cars. Parents tried to move us to a park a block away. Eventually we got older and accepted more space. This was the place that imbedded most of the values I hold today.

Our house was a five-room bungalow with attic-expansion space above the main-floor rooms. Five steps led up to the entry and living room, dining room, kitchen, two bedrooms, and one bath. Narrow stairways led up to an unfinished attic and down to a basement laundry, workroom, and a recreation room where my mother's brother, Chester Larson, lived until he joined the Army Signal Corps in 1941. My sister, Eileen, and I called this house our home until we left for college.

Our mother, Frances Elenore Larson Hanson, was energetic and capable in everything she did. She was born in 1911 in Minneapolis. Her father lost his foreman job building railroads to the Pacific Northwest when U.S. steel production was directed to WWI. The Larson family moved to an eighty-acre farm in Brunswick Township near Mora, Minnesota, in 1917 to be near her mother's Molin family.

Mother finished the country grade school two years early and graduated from Mora High School at sixteen. She played on the girls' basketball team and traveled with the boys' team to play in regional towns on cold winter nights. She was the first to attend college in her family, completing a degree in medical technology at the University of Minnesota before her twentieth birthday. She then went to work in a doctor's office in Duluth, Minnesota. When she and Dad married in Brunswick in 1934, she gave up her career to meet the cultural expectations of married women during the economic depression of the 1930s. Jobs were to be taken by those who needed family income, largely married men and single women. Later she said not continuing her professional career was her biggest disappointment. She did retrain herself at the university when her children were no longer coming home for lunch. Mother went back to work and job-shared a medical-technology position in a physician's office until she and Dad sold the house and moved to New Jersey in 1960.

Our father was Arthur E. Hanson. He was the sixth child, and the letter E was listed as his middle name when his home-birth in 1902 was recorded months later at the Kanabec County courthouse. When he was baptised at the Brunswick Immanuel Lutheran Church, his middle name became Emmanuel, in recognition of the church's name. His family changed the spelling from Hebrew to a Romanized version to fit his birth certificate.

Dad was tall and athletic and brought farmhand skills to urban life. He loved to make or fix things. He found any puzzle engaging. His workshop always had some project he was working on. At 6 foot 3 and 210 pounds he was my role model. He was forty years old in 1942, beyond draft or enlistment age. When he was identified as pre-diabetic about the same time, he lost twenty-five pounds, which he kept off for the rest of his life, and never developed active diabetes.

FIFTEENTH AND FIFTY-THIRD

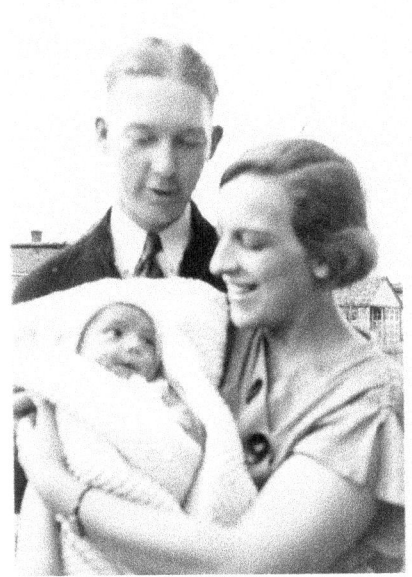 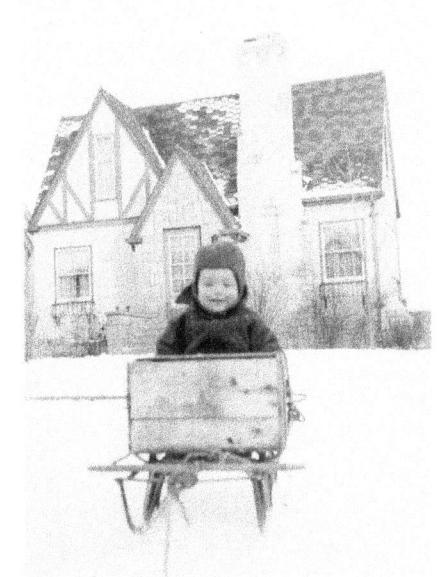

Left: Mother and Dad with me at four weeks old, April 1937
Right: In front of our house in the winter of 1938

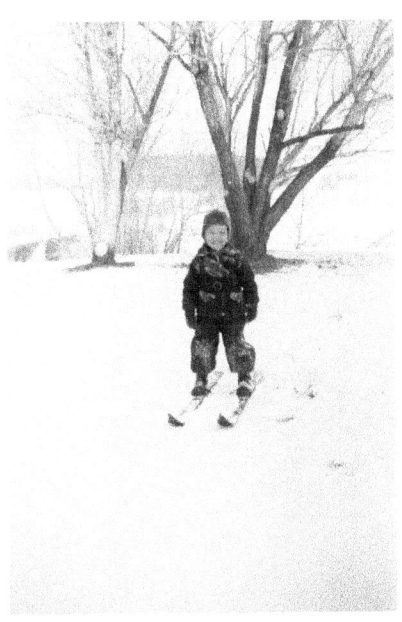

Third winter

Dad had an old first-baseman's glove in the basement. As soon as I could throw a ball, we played catch, and he took me to the park at the end of our street to teach me how to spin the ball to make it curve. When I had trouble hitting, he said, "If you can catch a ball, you can hit it." Later I learned he was the star first-baseman on a team from Braham, Minnesota, that won a state championship in 1928.

I was four years old in 1941 when my sister, Eileen Elenore, was born. I didn't understand what was happening or how my home was about to change. While Mother was in the hospital, a relative tried to restrain me as I fought off a bath that I didn't think I needed. I got out of her arms, but hit my head on the bathroom wall, leaving a dent that remained throughout my childhood.

Eileen and I got along unusually well for siblings, although I teased her regularly. In the neighborhood she was often referred to as "Stuie's little sister," which followed her into high school even after I left for college. She was limber, often doing headstands, splits, and cartwheels that I could never master. Both of us found school interesting and sought to do well, although the source of our motivation remains a mystery. Our parents were encouraging and always supported our activities, but I never felt they pushed us into doing things in which we had little interest.

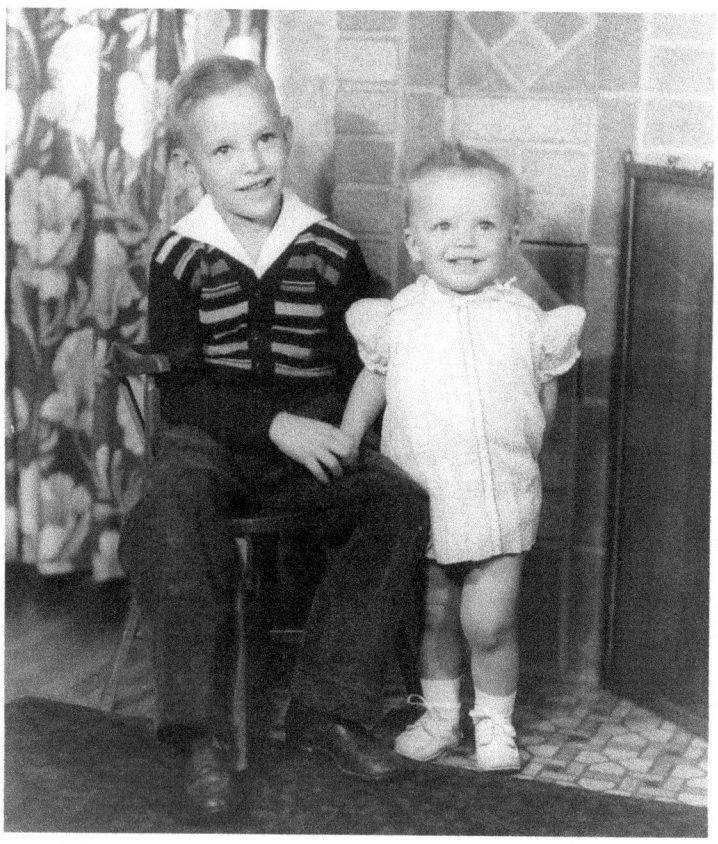

Eileen and me in our living room, December 1942

We spent six days a week with school and work. On Sunday mornings we attended a Swedish Lutheran church called Messiah Lutheran about five miles away. Dad's sisters, Ida and Hilda, were also members. Sunday school was held in a nearby late-nineteenth-century mansion with classes scattered throughout its many rooms. I must have been a problem because my parents were notified once that I was not to come the following week unless I could behave. When I was to start confirmation classes as a seventh grader, we moved to Diamond Lake, another Swedish Lutheran church, so I could walk to class after school.

This was the white middle-class neighborhood in which Eileen and I grew into our teens. A policeman (the boys liked the squad car he parked in the street), a barber, a plumber, a manufacturing manager, and a bass player for the Minneapolis Symphony were our neighbors. There were many Scandinavians, mostly Swedish, living in two-parent households with one to ten children. The closest neighbors were the Westlunds, Nelsons, and Johnsons. The Nelsons were Catholic and had ten kids. The Westlunds and Johnsons were Swedish Lutherans.

I believe place had a lot to do with the formation of my values and beliefs. Our parents and neighbors taught us the importance of education and work. Our parents created a home that was stable physically, financially, and emotionally. Eileen and I were fortunate and remain forever thankful for the positive upbringing we received in south Minneapolis in the 1940s and '50s. However, I did have some hard lessons to learn.

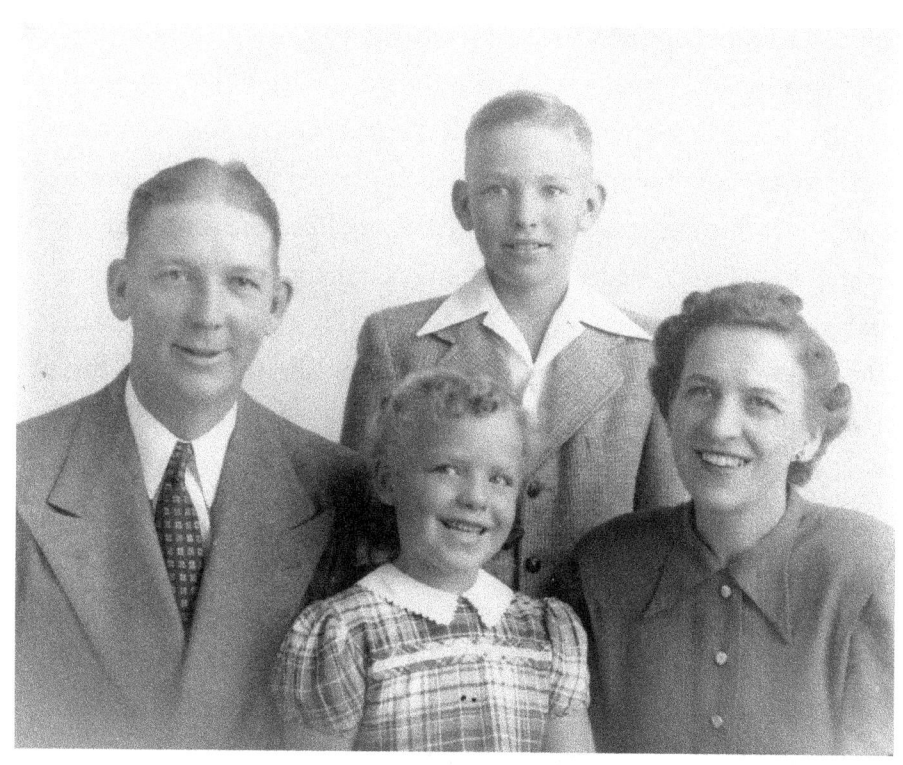

Our family in 1948

CHAPTER TWO

Lessons from Lying

I learned one of those lessons in third grade. Nathan Hale Grade School was three short blocks from our house. Most students walked back and forth twice a day. Stay-at-home mothers provided lunch or arranged for neighbors to manage the noon meals for their children when they were away.

For some reason, Chuckie took a disliking to me. I didn't taunt him, and I was too small to threaten him physically. He was in my third-grade classroom but was a year older after being held back the previous year. He persistently attacked me that winter for reasons that remain unclear to me.

At first Chuckie wrestled me into a snowbank as we walked along the same sidewalk going home for lunch or after school. I was taller but skinny and weak, and so not a physical match.

He began to stalk me. I would try to avoid him by taking alternate routes to and from school. He learned my deviations and frequently found me. I started to cut through neighbors' yards to avoid his assaults. When he caught me, he relished putting snow down my neck.

I was embarrassed and reluctant to tell anyone what was happening. I was cutting through neighbors' yards, often climbing snowbanks next to cleared walks. I dragged some snow back onto the sidewalks. One homeowner eventually called my parents to complain.

I knew about the boy who cried wolf and about Pinocchio, whose nose grew when he didn't tell the truth. But I had no direct personal connection to those stories. That was about to change.

When Dad came home from work and took me aside before dinner, I knew I was in trouble. When he asked if I knew about our neighbor's complaint, I denied that it was me who had messed his sidewalk. I said that it must have been someone else. Dad gave me several chances to confess before telling me the neighbor had followed me home and positively identified me.

I then told Dad everything — all about Chuckie's bullying that led to my shortcut routes and my inability to defend myself. What followed was not punishment but a serious discussion about the importance of always telling the truth.

Dad then called Chuckie's parents and told them the whole story. The bullying stopped immediately. Chuckie kept his distance and issued no more threats. A few weeks later I was surprised to be invited to his birthday party. I picked out an Army surplus backpack I thought he might like and, with some trepidation, attended the party. I was pleased to be welcomed and accepted as a friend. We had no further negative encounters, but never became close friends.

Why do these events remain in my mind seventy years later? There were other childhood events that affected my future, but I think these were especially significant. Communicating openly, being honest, and telling the truth are essential to building trust with others, and, in my case, with patients. Secondly, confronting an abuser is difficult but necessary. My parents went to the source and changed Chuckie's behavior with his parents' help. That was not the case with an abusing youth coach.

CHAPTER THREE

Ball Sports

Boys growing up in south Minneapolis in the 1940s had open areas to play and roam, creeks and lakes to tame, but no organized team sports in elementary school. I grew up in an all-white neighborhood whose diversity was limited to Protestants, Catholics, and Jews. Swedish Lutherans were prominent. We all mixed at Edgewater Park, which was at the end of our block at Fifteenth Avenue and Fifty-Fourth Street near Lake Nokomis.

The park was a reclaimed marsh and surrounded the southwest corner of the lake. There was no improved playing field, no backstop for baseball, no goalposts for football or soccer, and no backboards with hoops for basketball. It was a grassy, open space that sometimes flooded after a heavy rain.

Each spring we crafted a baseball diamond near some high ground. Large oak trees gave shade in summer. A football field overlaid the summer field in the fall. Baseball bases were crafted from what we could find. We used a small board for first base. Second base was always a problem: some sticks, an old rag, or a piece of cardboard that always seemed to move just as a close play developed, which led to arguments rarely settled easily. Third base wasn't much of a problem since we rarely had close plays at third. Runners either didn't get that far or made it all the way home due to some fielding error.

Our home base was actually a hole! Rain would make the batting area muddy, and a six-inch hole was used for drainage. It started as a depression that filled with water, so we dug the hole deeper. Nobody really thought of this solution; it just happened to work, so we kept it. A small cardboard covered the hole, but we were careful not to step directly on it.

Games were organized by those who showed up after school or on weekends. There were no adults, no leagues, no coaches, and no parents.

In the winter, skis, toboggans, and skates were our equipment. The sliding hills on Fourteenth and Seventeenth avenues along Minnehaha Creek have become much smaller since the 1940s. A warming house on Lake Nokomis provided a place to thaw out between hockey and red-rover games.

On the Nathan Hale Grade School grounds on Fifty-Fourth Street between Twelfth and Thirteenth avenues, there was one backstop for softball. The sixth graders held the franchise. The rest of us made up diamonds or kicked and ran with a soccer ball from one street across the play yard to the other in a game that melded football and soccer. We used the curbs as goal lines and chased scoring balls into the street.

There were no indoor basketball courts to use at any time of the year for pickup games. The school gym was used for physical education classes, but was otherwise closed. There were no elementary teams or leagues. I did have a basket in our driveway. A cement retaining wall on the left and a large poplar tree and neighbor's fence on the right narrowed the court. Rebounds to either side required a fence vault or a jump onto the sloping yard for retrieval. Cold weather required mittens that reduced our accuracy.

This was my athletic background as I entered seventh grade in 1949. Jack Marton, a former high-school athletic standout, was the volunteer neighborhood football coach who prepared boys for Washburn High School teams. He held forth at Pearl Park, another reclaimed marsh near Diamond Lake. It was closer to Ramsey Junior High and Washburn and ten blocks from our home on Fifteenth Avenue.

Coach Marton lived a block from my house and frequently offered me rides home. He was muscular and could demonstrate with accuracy the sport technique he was trying to teach. His dark hair, mature physique, and athletic ability made him our role model. He spoke with authority and had the respect of his players. I never learned if parents or former players gave him support other than their used equipment. As far as I know, he coached for the love of athletics and the success of his players.

By the time I showed up as a seventh grader, teams were already practicing. Coach Marton looked me over and asked how much I weighed. That's when I learned football teams were categorized by weight. As a skinny, five-foot-six specimen, I didn't show much promise.

"Go over to that black car and find some pads, a helmet, and shoes that fit. Come back, and we'll see what you can do," Coach said.

In the back seat of an old, black Studebaker sedan was a pile of pads and well-used pants and jerseys. The trunk was filled with cleated shoes. I found a pair of pants, helmet, shoulder, and hip pads, but no shoes that fit — I never did get football shoes that season.

"OK, Hanson, get in the line for head-on tackling." What had I gotten into? The first runner was Ronnie White. He was a year older and a lot bigger. Two missed tackles brought frowns from the coach and smiles from players waiting in line. Somehow I survived the tackling and blocking practices, but was not judged to be a "skilled position player." I was destined to be hidden somewhere in the offensive and defensive lines.

Games were played at night at Nicollet Field — later renamed Martin Luther King Jr. Field. The lights were dim and the well-used field could be dusty in dry weather and muddy after rains. I still did not have shoes with cleats. High-top farm boots didn't grip well. The lineman next to me was named an all-star, and I was an also-ran at the end of the season. I blamed my shoes.

Thus began my introduction to organized team sports and coaches. Football in the fall, basketball during the winter, and baseball each spring. Later in that first football season, another volunteer coach joined Coach Marton. I will call him Coach Pfahl. He seemed to know less about teaching basic skills and mostly took direction from Marton.

Coach Pfahl was different. He had balding hair, was not athletic appearing, had a slight abdominal paunch, and we were not told about any of his athletic accomplishments. He rarely tried to demonstrate specific techniques, and when he did, it was clear his skill-set did not match that of Coach Marton.

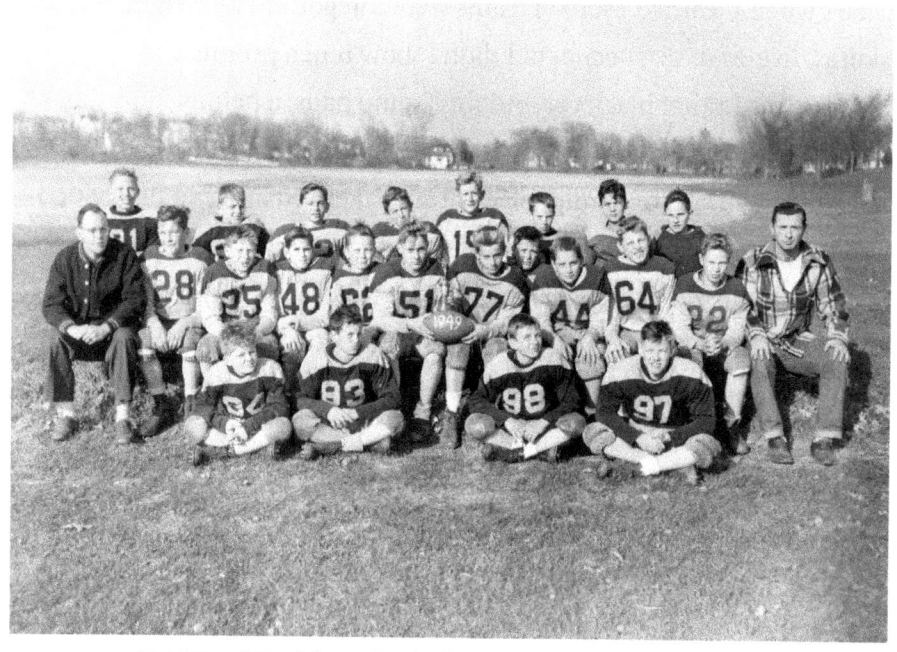

1949 Pearl Park boys football team. Coach Marton on the the right, Coach Pfahl on the left. I am behind Coach Pfahl (#91).

BALL SPORTS

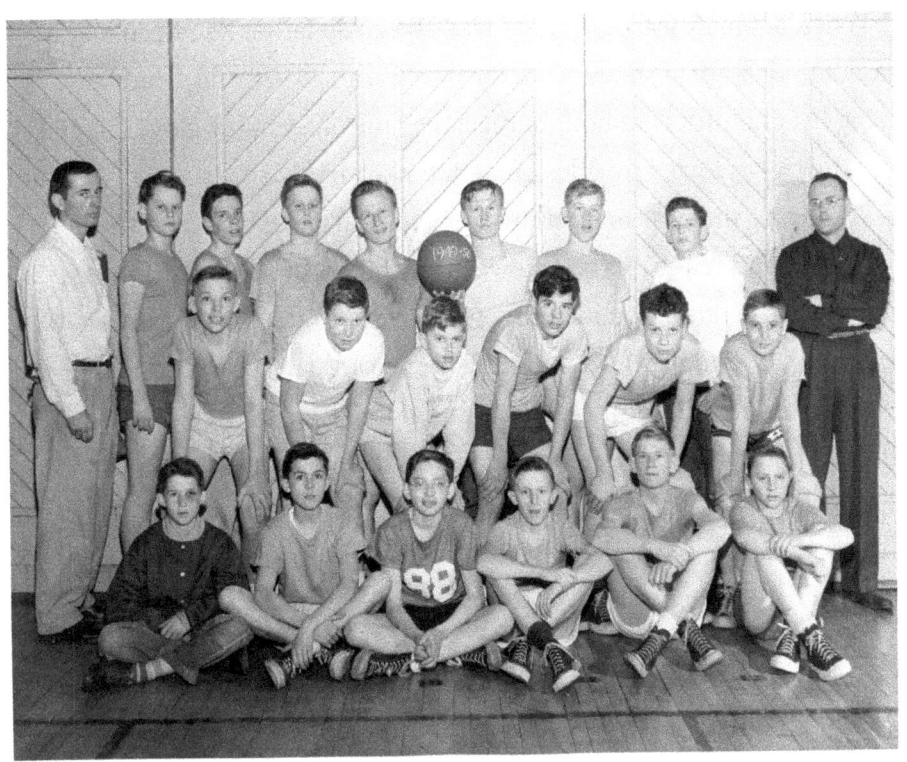

1949–50 basketball team. Coach Marton on the left, Coach Pfahl on the right. I am in the middle row far left.

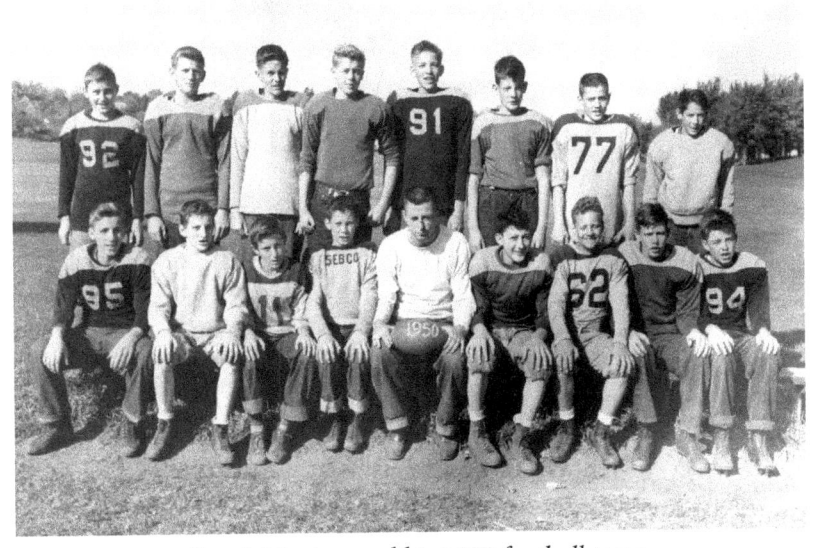

*Coach Marton and his 1950 football team
I am #91 right behind the coach.*

When baseball season came, I was eager. My father had been a first baseman on a town state championship team in 1928 and I had been using his old mitt. Dad bought me a new first-baseman's glove. Since I had the right glove, I was designated to play first base.

Our first game was on Lynnhurst Field near Lake Harriet. It had backstops and real bases tied down with spikes. I was issued a heavy wool uniform and I bought shoes with cleats. In the first game I had four hits (two singles, a triple, and a home run), almost hitting for "the cycle" (a single, double, triple, and home run) in a single game. The game and my hits were written up in the neighborhood paper. I thought I was destined for stardom.

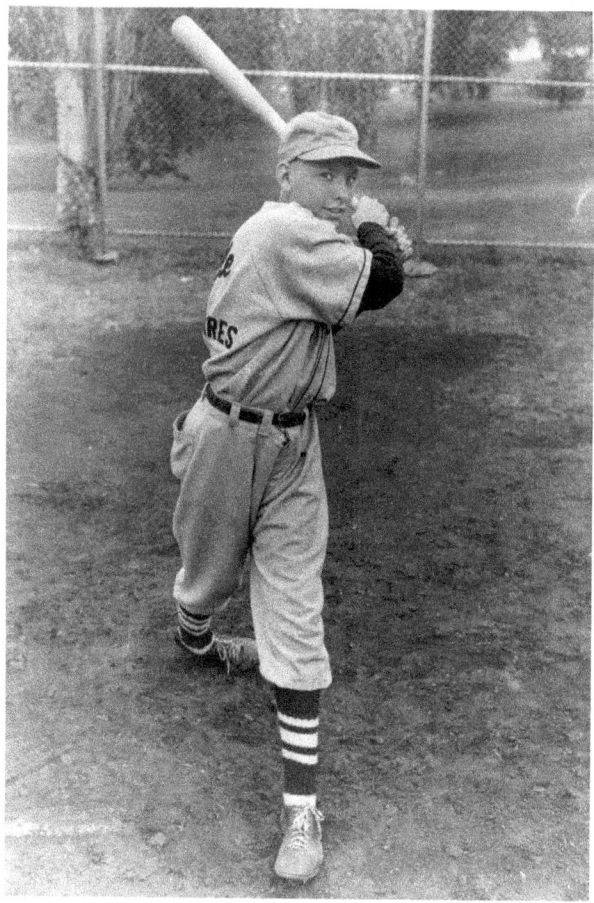

Seventh grade, age thirteen

Our team was winning and leading the league. One Friday toward the end of the season my mother said, "Stuart, your game tomorrow has been canceled." Taken aback, I asked why. "I can't tell you, but the parents are meeting instead."

I was left home to wonder why. When my parents returned, I was all questions, but the only answer I received was that Mr. Pfahl would no longer be coaching us. It took me several weeks to find out that Coach Pfahl had been molesting one of my teammates. I heard this from a friend. No adult ever addressed the issue with me. Jack Marton continued coaching, but one of our players was missing for the rest of the season. As far as I know, the police were never notified and there was no further investigation or explanation.

Twenty-seven years later in 1977, our son, Peter, was on the Lynnhurst Field traveling basketball team. Guess who was coaching? The team was technically called Washburn Traveling Team and was sponsored by the Minneapolis Park Board, but Mr. Pfahl was the coach and the players called it "Pfahl's Team." He was well ensconced and revered by players and current parents. I had a talk with Peter, Coach Pfahl, and several parents. No one knew of any inappropriate behavior by Pfahl. He knew I remembered his past. What more should I do? Raise a 27-year-old issue that others were denying? I chose to let Peter play and to keep vigilant. As far as I know, there were no further incidents of abuse, but I remained wary until I heard that he had died years later.

As I contemplated writing these memoirs, I wondered how, or even if, I should write about this experience. Neither I nor my son were molested. Sixty-seven years had passed, and the involved player and coach have died. But the issues of child abuse and sexual molestation are relevant. Many adults in power positions are still sexually molesting minors. The most prominent and egregious have been priests in the Roman Catholic Church. The church covered up the issues internally much like our parents did in 1950. Sexual-abuse laws were present in mid-twentieth century, but community norms sent the issue underground. Unfortunately, some of those attitudes still persist.

During a fifty-fifth Washburn High School reunion in 2015, I discussed our experience and the parents' handling of our problem coach with some of the team members. They all said I should write about it. Then one of our star players said, "He abused me, too. I never told my parents or anyone else until about two years ago."

I was startled, but when I thought about it, our parents' response had been usual for the time and unfortunately similar responses are all too frequent today. Many young people are not aware of what constitutes inappropriate touching, and those affected can be too embarrassed to report it to an adult they trust. Many adults do not know what to do or are reluctant to make a formal complaint to the police. Law enforcement officers are reluctant to bring cases to trial where the evidence is not rock solid. Child abuse remains a public health problem that developed countries have not solved. The children of today and tomorrow deserve better.

CHAPTER FOUR

Who Do You Want to Be?

When I misbehaved as a young boy, Dad would say, "You need to practice being a man; someday you will be grown up and you won't know it."

My father's sisters, Ida and Hilda, and his brother Carl were always probing me. What did I want to do for work? Baseball player was not an acceptable response. They were looking for something more. Years later I realized they were also asking, "Who do you want to be? What will be your character?"

Ida and Hilda were born on a small hand-tilled farm in northern Sweden called a "torp." They had immigrated to the United States as children with their parents and settled in the community of Brunswick, north of Minneapolis, in 1900. They finished eighth grade in the local country school and went to work to support themselves and to help their younger siblings get more education. Along with their older sister, Margaret, they supported a future engineer (my father), a future physician (Uncle Carl), and a future social worker (Aunt Bertha) during their high school, college, and graduate-school years. Single in midlife, Ida and Hilda closely followed their nieces' and nephews' education.

They were always interested in our development. All of us knew that when we saw them, we would have to answer their questions about school, about our classes, how we were doing, and what we were planning to do with our lives.

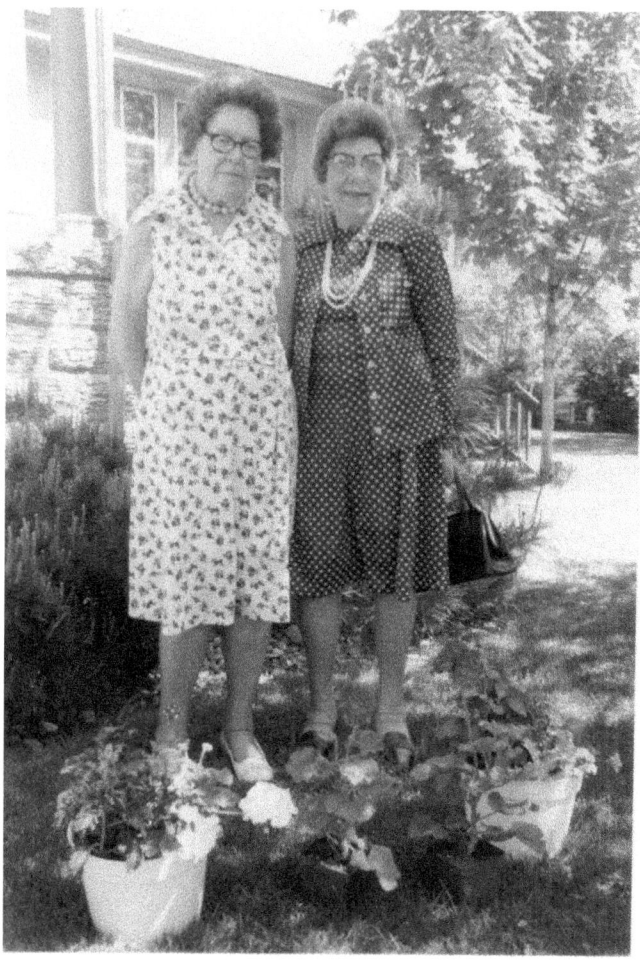

Aunt Ida and Aunt Hilda, 1978

I believe their concern for our futures helped me consider choosing a medical career. I can't say when I began thinking seriously about medicine. Since my father and my mother's brother, Chester, were electrical engineers, I was exposed to electricity and its principles at an early age. We made working telephones from leftover parts. An old magneto connected to a lightbulb burned brightly, as long as someone turned the crank. In fifth grade I actually made a motor out of five large nails, a thin wire, a fishing cork, and some glass tubing. My motor earned second-place in a citywide science competition. I was disappointed. I thought my work should have been first.

It was my father's brother, Uncle Carl, who had the most influence on my choice of career. He was a physician who, in the 1930s, limited his practice to children before there was formal training in pediatrics. He completed medical school at the University of Minnesota in 1929, bought a Ford Model-T, and with other graduates, drove to their internships in Hackensack, New Jersey. A nurse at the hospital, Marion Weil, from Long Island found him interesting. When they married, they settled permanently in Cranford, New Jersey. She had agreed to move west from Long Island, but not as far west as Minnesota.

Each summer Carl and Marion would arrive by train at the Milwaukee Depot in Minneapolis for their annual visit to the prairie province and farm where the Hanson family grew up. The Minnesota relatives would anticipate their visit for months. Marion accepted her Minnesota family and tolerated the annual visits. But Carl was back in his element, meeting old friends, reconnecting with family, and fishing whenever he had an opportunity. The Hanson family came from Sweden in 1900 with five children. My father was the first to be born in the United States, followed by Carl and their baby sister, Bertha, who was the eighth and last in line. She was accepted to medical school in the 1930s when female students were a small minority of physicians. Her economic situation and lack of medical-school encouragement led her away from medicine into a successful career as a social worker and a writer.

One of Uncle Carl's obligations to all the young mothers in the family was examining their children during his stay. These visits were held at one of the family farms in Brunswick during a Sunday. After a big noon meal, he would set up in a parlor or bedroom, close the door, and he would have private conversations and perform physical exams with each child. Then our mothers would be called in individually, and Carl would give them his assessment. One year I was advised to take more cod-liver oil for vitamin C during the winter. Another year I needed arch supports and shoes that were certainly not stylish in grade school. Did we fear our soft-spoken, fatherly, pipe-smoking uncle? Maybe a little. But we also held him in high regard as did our parents. He also asked us, "What do you want to do when you grow up?"

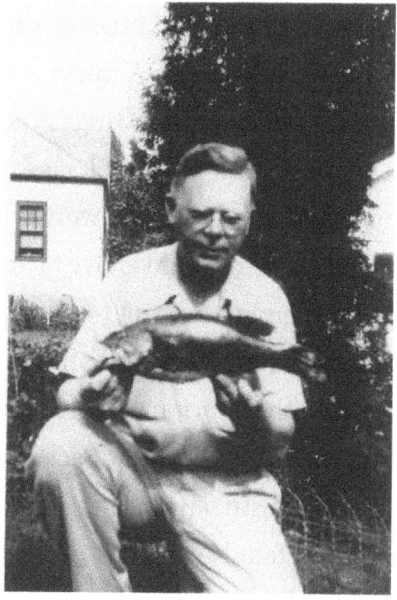

Uncle Carl in 1944 with his catch of the day

Our house in Minneapolis had a basement workshop. My father could fix almost anything and create something out of whatever material was available. I was four when the United States entered World War II. The following years brought food and gas rationing, clean-plate clubs, and fear of invasion. Consumer items were scarce, and no cars were being produced. Our new black, sleek, 1941 Buick sedan was sold for a nice profit, and we drove a 1934 Packard for the rest of the war years. Bicycles, wagons, and other toys were leftovers from the 1930s. I had my own small workbench and beginner tools, but soon learned to use full-size saws, drills, and hammers, and graduated to Father's big bench. I made workable telephones out of spare parts, connected magnetos to lightbulbs, rebuilt electric trains, and created things out of wood.

In sixth grade Miss Woods had us review various occupations. Some parents also talked to us about their jobs. In truth I don't remember the day, but Mike Bentsen, a sixth-grade classmate, told me this story sixty-five years later. As a climax to the subject, the teacher went around the room asking each of us what we wanted to be. Mike, being early in the alphabet, said, "I want to be a cowboy." The next boy said, "I want to be a fireman." Mike thought silently, "I wish I had thought of that." According to Mike, when it was my turn I said I wanted to be a physician. Miss Woods said, "That's wonderful," and effusively congratulated me.

What I do remember, however, was a class project in Miss Mehalek's eighth-grade social studies class. We started with a personal-interest-and-preference test. This predated Myers-Briggs testing and the Minnesota Multiphasic Personality Inventory. We answered the questions on our multiple-choice survey by making a pinprick in one of five columns. Among the teenage boys it quickly became known as "The Prick Test." The semi-thick paper with a series of holes was scored by a light-reader.

My preferences were in two categories: scientific or social-related careers. The careers listed in the first category were scientist, engineer, mathematician, researcher, inventor, physician. In the second category were salesman, businessman, social worker, nurse, teacher. (Notice how "man" was used for sales and business while social worker, nurse, and teacher, by implication, might be suitable for girls.)

I decided it was time to explore engineering. Dad had exposed me to electrical engineering. Civil engineering wasn't attractive to me, but aeronautical engineering was. At the time in 1950, before Sputnik, satellites, and space stations, this seemed to be a dynamic area with lots of future prospects. I had only watched airplanes, and no one in our family had ever been inside one, let alone flown.

I studied the aerodynamics of flight and the challenges of space. I studied how these large machines were held in the air by a relative vacuum over the wings or by the thrust of rockets yet to be built.

There was excitement in the classroom as one by one we made oral presentations to our classmates and our watchful teacher. My report was filled with diagrams of planes, rockets, and the dynamics of flight. Miss Mehalek, a four-foot-eleven, sturdy, demanding, dynamo of a teacher, had encouraging things to say when I finished. Then she added, "So you want to be an aerospace engineer. You could be a good one."

I was still interested in medicine when we started this project, but I had wanted to explore an engineering field to test my commitment. I responded to her question with, "No. I want to be a physician."

She looked shocked. Everyone laughed, and it took a while for the class to settle down before going onto the next presentation.

That was the first time I personally remember going public with my thoughts of becoming a physician. From then on I selected courses in high school and college to fit a medical track. I did play games with friends, telling them I was going to take wildlife management at Montana State. I may have told Ida and Hilda that once or twice. But my medical-technologist mother, Uncle Carl, and my engineer father never doubted what I wanted to do if I had the opportunity.

It was at Dartmouth College, after leaving home and realizing I might be able to make it into medical school, that I began to think about "Who did I want to be?" as opposed to "What did I want to do?" I wasn't thinking much about how I affected others during the first years of college. I made jokes easily, did goofy stuff at times, but was perceived as a serious student. For some reason I thought saying "Fine," when someone asked

"How are you?" was superfluous. I began responding with one word, "Functioning." Or, if I wanted to be more effusive, I would say, "I guess I'm functioning." This went on for a few weeks before Henry Hoff, an upper-class fraternity brother, took me aside in the Beta Fraternity House library and asked why I was responding in this way. Was I depressed? When I assured him I was just fooling around, he said, "Well, you're making the rest of us depressed, and we would like you to stop."

That's when I began thinking about how I affected others and how I related to them even on a superficial level. I decided to adopt a positive attitude, be more friendly, and become an optimist. I started to make eye contact and greet everyone I passed on campus. Nobody complained again. The next year I was elected president of the Dartmouth Lutheran Club and invited to run for senior class president, which I declined because I was starting medical school. The next year I was elected president of Alpha Kappa Kappa, Dartmouth's only medical fraternity.

It was much later that I learned about method acting — how by taking on the actions of a character, you become that person. The popular business lessons of the 1990s, taken from the Seattle Fish Market about choosing your attitude and being present when relating to others, came later. Being more optimistic was more fun and people seemed to like me better. Years later I summarized these ideas in what I call an operating principle, "You are what you do." For now I'll say, "My glass is more than half full, but I'm careful not to break the glass."

CHAPTER FIVE

Immigrant Farms

My Hanson grandparents emigrated from Sweden to Minnesota. Hans Abraham and Anna Karolina had five children when they came from a small hamlet called Seljon (pronounced sell-yon) in northern Sweden in 1900. Their economic prospects in the late nineteenth century in Sweden were poor.

Hans Abraham's mother, Maria Katrina, my great-grandmother, came from a family that owned farm-and-timber land in Ångermanland near the city of Sollefteå, Sweden. Her family was considered wealthy. The oldest son was set to inherit the farm, and the daughters were expected to marry sons of landowners. But Maria married Hans Abraham, my great-grandfather, who was an outgoing farmhand with no prospects of inherited land. I've been told he was an excellent singer, played several instruments, and livened up most parties.

When Maria married Hans, her family disinherited her. The new couple was given ten acres of land, called a torp, which was to return to Maria's family in fifty years. My great-grandparents had a family of five daughters and one son, my grandfather, who was also named Hans Abraham. The operation of the small hand-tilled farm could be passed down to the eldest son, but only for the remaining years left on the lease.

Another major problem was that the land was insufficient to support a family. Their small farm would soon go back to its original owners. Their prospects were to serve others, either in an owner's house, in their fields, or in their woods.

The concept of "Almans Lan" was developing in Sweden, which meant all of Sweden belonged to everyone. A Swedish citizen could stay one day on any private or public land, then had to move on. For a young couple this was not enough time to build a shelter, till the soil, and raise a family.

Anna Karolina's parents and brother had migrated to Brunswick, Minnesota, ten years earlier. Nearby land, available for homesteading, was waiting for the expanding family. They sold their livestock, most of their possessions, bought passage to America, packed up the family, and began to say their good-byes. Can you imagine leaving your home, your extended family, your friends, your country, and your citizenship for a new life in a foreign country you had never visited? Prospects for reuniting with anyone left behind were remote. Hans, Sr. could not bear to see his only son's family the day they left. He later wrote a touching letter apologizing for not being there to say good-bye. That letter is a family treasure that has been read at all subsequent family reunions in the United States.

When my great-grandparents died in Sweden, Maria was buried in her family's churchyard plot. Hans did not earn an individual site, had no permanent marker, and the only record we have is a church book that states he died "ut fatig," which means "penniless."

The sixty-acre farm in Brunswick Township, Minnesota, must have been a welcome change from their ten-acre torp in Sweden. Family members helped cut logs for their home and barn. Fields were opened after cutting the trees and grubbing out the remaining stumps. Chickens and pigs were bought and penned, and cows were pastured. When they got a horse they began to feel established in their new country. Most fieldwork was by hand. A hand-planter was still in use when I was growing up in the 1940s.

The planter had a long wooden handle with a V-shaped box on its end held together by a spring. Corn seeds or a piece of potato were placed in the shaped container, which was driven into the ground with a foot to make a hole. Then the handle was moved to open the box and drop the seeds. When the planter was removed from the ground, the spring closed the box, and the planter was ready for more seeds and another hole. When I was old enough to work in the fields, I was given a planter to help my dad and Uncle Albert (whom everybody called "Happy") plant corn and potatoes. The Hanson homestead was a subsistence farm in the process of being mechanized.

By the time I was around the farm in the 1940s, the log house had been expanded, sheeted with clapboard outside, and plastered inside to look like any farmhouse built in the 1920s. The barn was also covered with milled-wood siding. A second barn for horses, a granary and machine shed, and a summer kitchen built with framing lumber completed the farmstead. Did I mention the outhouse conveniently situated behind the machine shed? (Inside plumbing wasn't installed until the mid-1950s.)

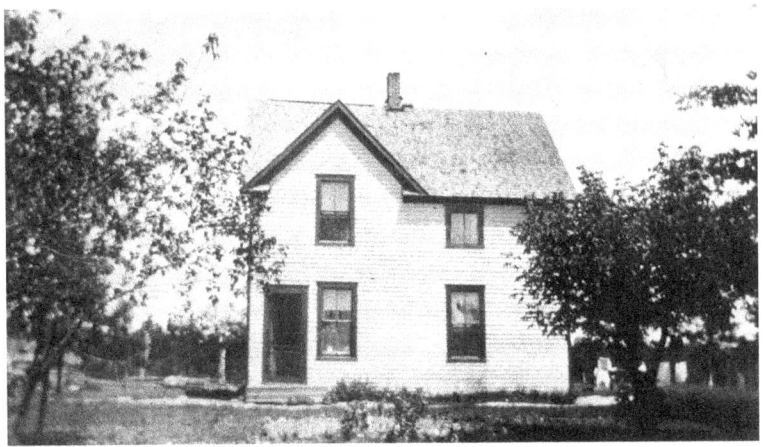

The Hanson farmhouse after siding was applied to the original logs

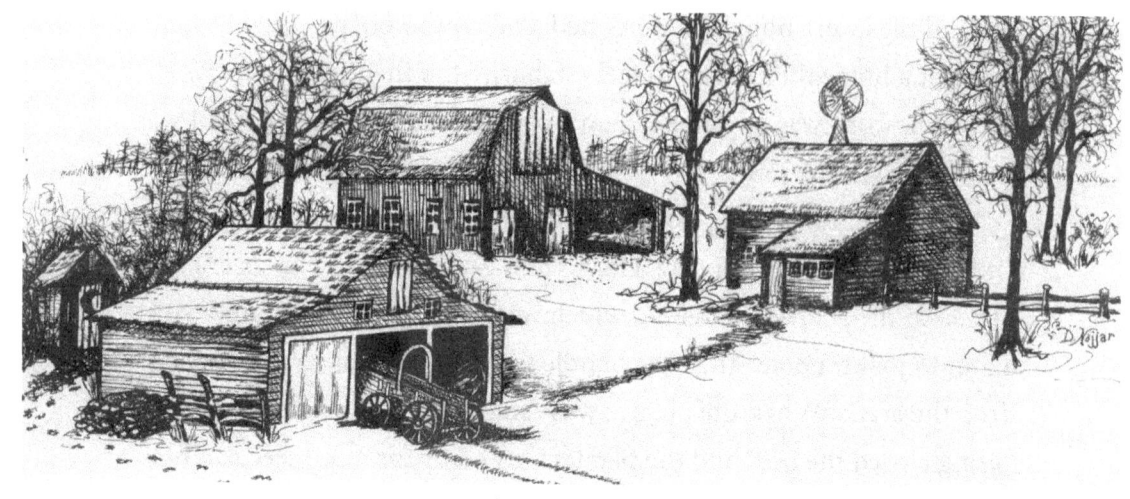

*The Hanson farm outbuildings as sketched
by my cousin Dee Anne Nygren Najjar*

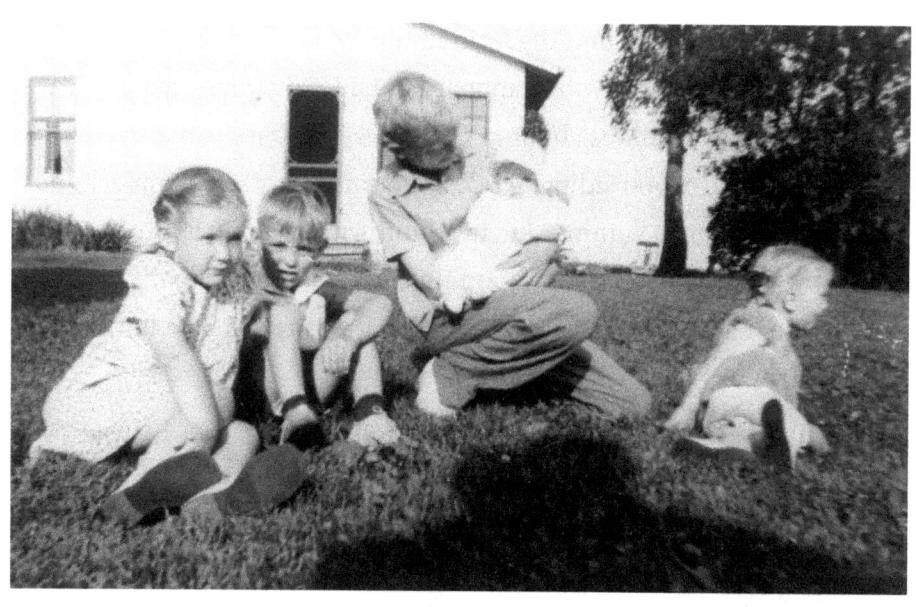

*The Hanson grandchildren, 1941
Left to right: Marion Lovas (Held), me, Bob Hanson,
my sister Eileen Hanson-Kelly in Bob's arms, and Dee Anne Nygren (Najjar)*

Kerosene lamps provided evening and morning light in the house and barns. On Christmas Eve there was always a candle in the window, visible from the road, to light the way. After we had Christmas Eve dinner and presents at the nearby Larson farm, our family would head into the cold night to drive the mile and a half to the Hanson farm. My sister and I were happy to see the window candle casting light across the snowy field.

The Hanson grandparents, aunts, uncles, and cousins would have eaten, and they would be waiting to light the tree and wait for Santa. Candles on the tree were carefully lit, and the children were kept at a safe distance as we sang carols. When the candles burned down under careful watch, they were extinguished as we heard reindeer stomping on the roof. We knew that Santa would soon appear and begin distributing packages. As the years passed we thought the tall Santa one year looked a lot like my father. Another year, Santa's girth seemed to resemble Uncle Happy.

Electricity finally came to the farm after WW ll (about 1950), when the government-subsidized Rural Electrification Association strung lines to "unelectrified" parts of the township.

Grandmother Hanson was short and had grey hair by the time I knew her. She did her cooking on a woodstove that also heated the two-story house in the winter. During the summer she moved to a summer kitchen in a smaller well-ventilated building nearby. (They also sometimes slept in the cooler building.) Grandma's Swedish rye bread was a hoped-for delicacy when anyone visited. Her hand-knit hats, mittens, and socks were frequent Christmas presents; I still have one sock and a pair of mittens.

Grandpa Hanson had severe arthritis and walked with two canes that I liked to play with as a small child. There are movies showing me pulling at his canes and making him even more unsteady. He was another Hanson who was always interested in what I was doing and what I was planning to do with my life. His field days were mostly over except as a supervisor, but when milking time came, he picked up a pail and headed to the barn.

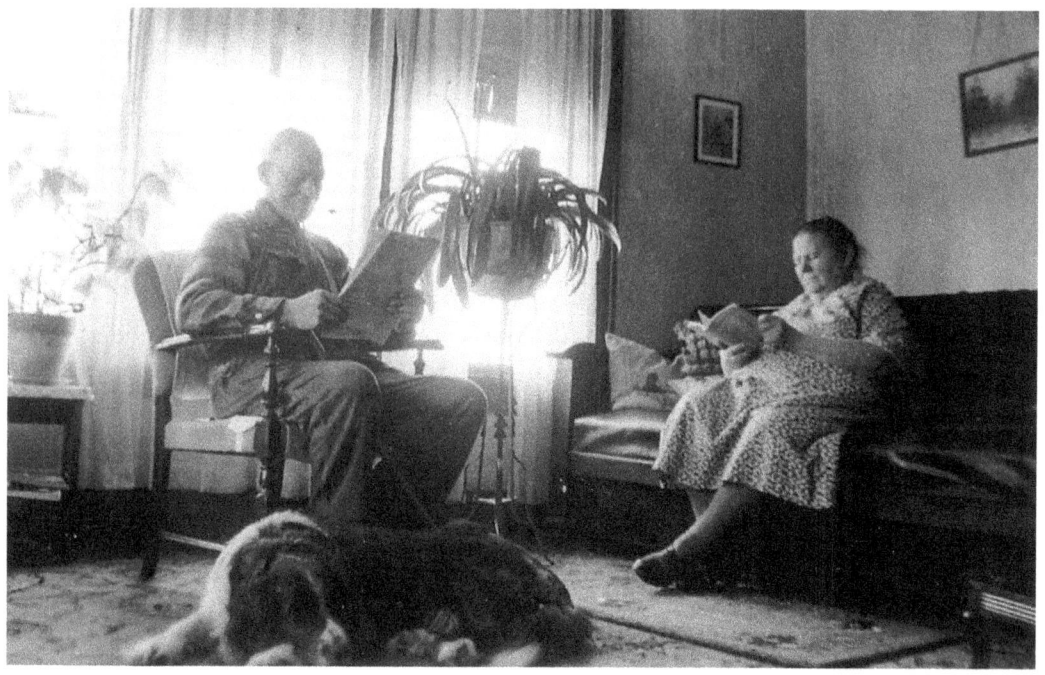

Grandma and Grandpa Hanson with their dog Pal in their living room, 1941

The pasture still had a few trees, but was mostly open grassland. A windmill drew water for the animals. A large orchard with "eating apples" and "baking apples" was at the back of the house. What wasn't eaten in the fall was preserved in jars for the winter. A horse-drawn drill was used for planting oats and wheat. Milking was done by hand, and anyone available was enlisted to help. If you claimed you didn't know how, you were soon taught how to clean udders and rhythmically squeeze to fill your pail.

The Hanson homestead was a mile south of the Brunswick Immanuel Lutheran Church.

IMMIGRANT FARMS

A half mile east of the church was the Arvid and Ellen Larson farm. This was where my mother and her brother, Chester, grew up. Their family had moved from Minneapolis in 1917 to be near Grandmother Ellen's parents, who had sold their butcher shop in Minneapolis and moved to Brunswick Township several years earlier.

Why Ellen's parents (another set of great-grandparents), August and Allette Molin, made the move is unclear, but the Larsons had a significant reason. Arvid, who emigrated from Sweden with his older sister as a ten-year-old boy in 1890, had become a foreman on railroad crews building the Great Northern Railway through Montana. As the United States began diverting its steel production to support England at the beginning of World War I in 1914, steel was sent to Europe, and railroad construction was halted. Without a job and with a young daughter and son, my Larson grandparents moved to an established farm also in Brunswick, Minnesota. It was an eighty-acre farm with the Groundhouse River transecting its pasture. Fields led down to the river on both sides. A single barn held all the cattle, horses, and chickens. Pigs had their own pen and a straw-covered house. Pregnant sows were housed in a smaller shed connected to the corncrib.

A substantial granary had lean-to sheds on three sides for machinery. A separate shed was filled with sawdust and ice taken from a nearby lake each winter. The two-story farmhouse had a big kitchen with a woodstove and a large table for eating four times a day. A living room with a couch and Grandpa's desk connected to a dining room where the floor sagged about six inches, making a nice incline for a little boy's cars.

A front parlor held a bust of Shakespeare, portraits of parents, and any special furniture including Grandpa's big rocking chair and a leather settee. The room was rarely used except on Christmas Eve or after a Sunday dinner when the minister and his family came. Four bedrooms upstairs provided ample space for anyone bringing their families or friends for a visit. We still have the rocking chair.

There was no inside plumbing. My job as a child was to pump water from a well between the house and garage and bring the pail to Grandma's kitchen. The toilet was an outhouse attached to the barn backing up to the barn's manure pile. Some called it the library where Sears catalogues were stacked. There were four separate holes inside, including a small one for children. Women and children often used the facility at the same time, especially at night.

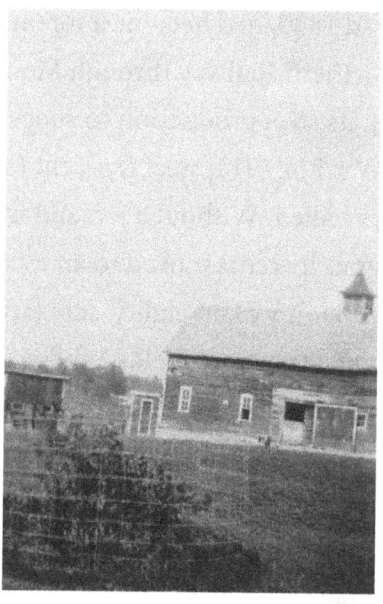

Sideview of the barn, attached "library," and pig house

The Larson eighty-acre farm was a step up from the Hanson farm, but still would be called a subsistence farm today. This was my Larson grandparents' home for thirty-four years and my country playground while I was growing up in the 1940s.

Grandma Larson was a vigorous woman. Her hair was brown and always well pinned or bobbed. She had her cows to milk and chickens to feed besides keeping house and making all the meals. Monday was washday, Tuesday she baked several kinds of bread, and Wednesday afternoon she either went to the ladies' aid society at the church or to town to sell eggs and get supplies.

She was the Brunswick Co-op Creamery's secretary. She added up the amount of milk and calculated the butterfat content each farmer delivered to the creamery. A day or two before payday, her adding machine sang into the night, and she wrote checks for delivery at the creamery on payday. It was not unusual to have another farmer's car drive up the curving road by the root cellar seeking an advance several days before checks were due.

Grandpa Larson was one of the more successful farmers in the area. He had strong ideas and expected young people like myself to accept his direction. I was accepting, but some of the neighbor boys were less compliant. He had great respect for his animals and treated them like a father. It was a sad day when a favorite animal was sent to market. When he took me to town he seemed proud to tell his friends, "This is my grandson."

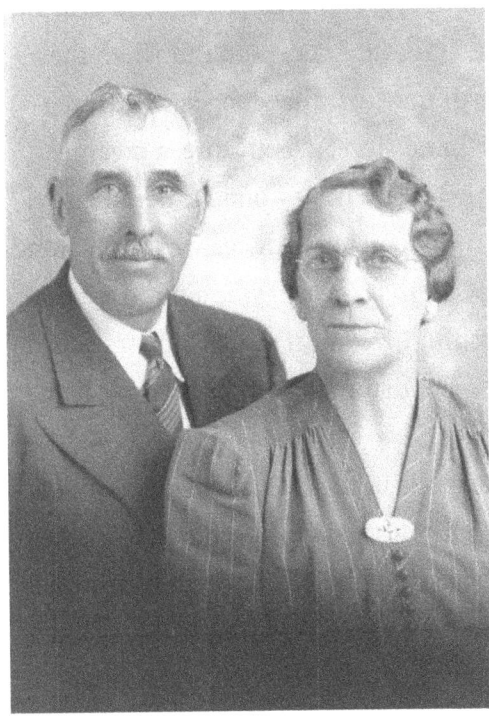

Grandma and Grandpa Larson on their twenty-fifth wedding anniversary, 1944

The chickens he raised were all Rhode Island Reds, a rust-colored breed that laid brown eggs. Grandpa liked me to go with him to the fields when I was small. I suppose he was getting me ready to be of help as I grew older. One day, when I was about five, I refused to go with him. The rooster had decided I was competition and would chase after me anytime I walked across the yard. Grandpa assured me that would not happen, and if it did, he would defend us with his large four-tined hay-pitching fork.

As we headed to the fields we passed the open chicken yard. The rooster saw me coming, lowered his head, and charged. "Here he comes," I yelled.

With one swoop, the fork came off Grandpa's shoulder and impaled the charging rooster, killing it on the spot. We had to delay our fieldwork, clean the chicken, and explain to Grandma why Sunday's dinner menu had changed.

Brunswick was a farming community mostly populated by Swedish immigrants. In the nineteenth century it was considered the logical site for a county seat, since it was near the county's center. But when the railroad was built seven miles north in Mora, the village growth stagnated. By the 1940s there was a general store, a feed store, a creamery, a two-room school, and two Swedish churches — one Lutheran and one Baptist. Each church had its own cemetery. An early sawmill along the Groundhouse River was gone. All that was left was a pond we used for winter skating and summer fishing. The local virgin pine trees had become houses, sheds, and barns. Their stumps were cleared for fields, pastures, and homesteads.

For a boy growing up in Minneapolis in the 1940s, having grandparents who lived on farms was not unusual. Having two farms to visit in the same area was. Having a river passing directly through your play yard was a magnet for cousins and playmates. Watching tadpoles turn into frogs was magical. Swimming in a gentle river current, chasing cows and horses, digging for summer ice in the icehouse, finding the nooks and crannies in the barn, picking eggs in the chicken coop, and swilling (feeding) the pigs were all part of a summer day.

Alfalfa hay and oats were the mainstay crops produced to feed the livestock. Hybridized corn also had a modest field position. A large vegetable garden with a long patch of rhubarb supplemented the family's meat and eggs.

Haying time was fun as a young boy, but became more work as I got older, taller, and stronger. A horse-drawn mower laid down the hay; so-called dump-rakes crossed the fields producing rows of collected hay for fieldworkers to form into rain-protected piles called cocks. Drying hay was always a problem. Weather interfered frequently making field decisions unpredictable. Having "hay down" always created anxiety until it was in a well-formed field stack or in the barn.

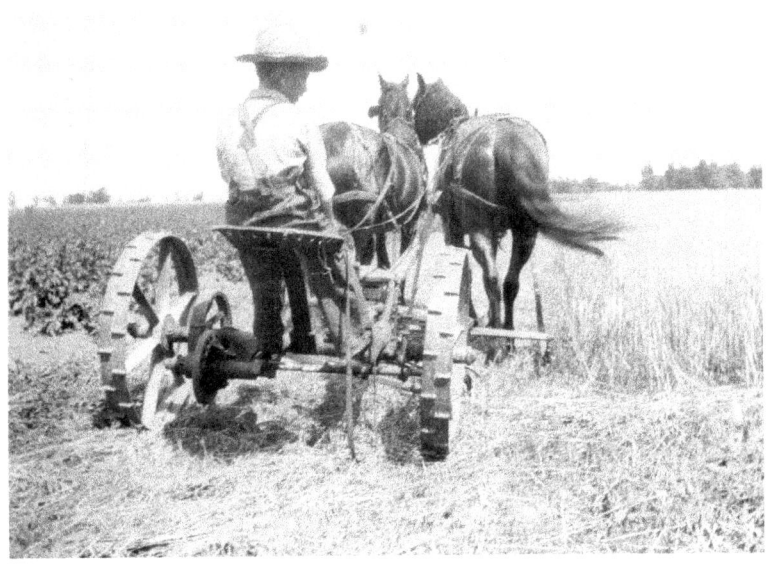

Me with King and Queen mowing hay, 1944

Getting hay into the barn was exciting. Haycocks from the field were hand-pitched onto a wagon rack pulled by two horses, called King and Queen, who did the heavy lifting and pulling. (Dick, the third horse, was used only when extra power was required.) When the hayrack was loaded, the horses moved it to a field stack or to the barn's hayloft doors.

At the barn my job was to unhook the horses, move them to the back of the barn, and attach the team to a hay rope connected by pulleys to a large fork plunged into a corner of the hay load in the front of the barn. At the call "All's ready," I drove the team away from the barn. Up rose the fork loaded with hay and down the center of the barn until I heard another call to stop after the hay fork had been tripped and the hay dumped. Then, I turned the horses around and pulled the rope back as another fork load of wagon hay was readied for lifting. Eventually the wagon was emptied, the horses were reattached to the wagon, and we headed back to the field for another load. Helping my grandfather and his workers was rewarding for a young boy who could now take his place at the table where the workers were fed.

Thrashing time was the summer highlight. Neighbors came together to help bring the grain harvest from field to granary. By the mid 1940s hand fieldwork was mostly replaced by horse-drawn machines on the Larson and Hanson farms. A grain binder pulled by King, Queen, and Dick, cut and bound the Larson grain in the field. Bundles were small enough to be handled by hand or pitchforks. Stacking bundles in large round stacks near farm buildings to be threshed later had been common. This allowed a hired threshing-machine operator to schedule threshing throughout the fall. By the time I was aware of farm practices, the Hanson farm still used this method. But, the Larson farm did what was called "shock threshing." Bundles of grain stalks were set up in the field in groups of twelve with the grain heads upright for rain protection and drying. Six neighboring farms joined together to move one farm's harvest from field to threshing machine to granary in the morning and they then all moved to the next farm in the afternoon.

Over the years my roles evolved from driving horses to driving grain trucks and eventually to manning a bundle wagon by myself. The last year on the farm I was designated to stack the straw. Straw was used for animal bedding in the barn and was stacked to cover the pigs' winter house near the barn. This was something Grandpa usually did. Dealing with straw and chaff coming directly out of the thresher was a dirty job. He wanted it stacked so it made a perfect dome over a wood-framed pigpen. I argued that I was more useful in the field or driving the grain truck, but he had his mind made up. Maybe he had decided he'd had enough of straw being blown in his face and down his neck while he sweated stacking straw into place on a hot humid day. As I struggled through the morning, I was thinking about our noon dinner, but when the time came, we hadn't finished, so the others all ate in shifts while threshing continued into the afternoon. Finally, Grandpa relieved me from this miserable job. That was my last day of threshing.

Another threshing day stands out above all others. I must have been eight, and I was not old enough to be of much use pitching bundles in the field or at the threshing machine. I could do some of the harnessing and driving the horses. Algot Ryberg was hired to work the Larson farm bundle-wagon. I bridled the horses, he harnessed them. We connected them to the wagon, and we were off across the bridge to a pair of fields north of the Groundhouse River. We were first in the field and started to load as I drove the horses from shock to shock.

Henry Holmberg arrived with his team and began loading near the entry gate. Down the road came Johnny Anderson casually waving a greeting. I turned to move our wagon to another row of shocks, when I heard a loud crash and saw the Anderson horses racing through the gate without Johnny. They hit the back of the Holmberg rack and kept running. Henry tried to hold his horses by their bridles, but they were also off and running. Two runaway teams were on the same field. Algot held the bridles of King and Queen. The bridle eye-blinders must have worked because our horses stayed in place as the other two teams raced away. When the Anderson team came to a fence separating two fields, they somehow wound up with one horse on each side. As the wagon parts went flying, fence posts and barbed wire went spiraling in the air. About a quarter mile of wire and wood was scattered in the fence line when they finally came to rest near the river's edge.

After being transfixed on the scene taking place, I looked for the Holmberg team. They were eating alfalfa in the next field, dragging what was left of the wagon. Henry was sitting on the ground holding the left side of his face. He had gone under his wagon after one of the horses stepped on his face. Johnny Anderson was lying motionless on the road. Very soon Grandma was in the '37 Dodge coming from the farmhouse across the river. She picked up the injured. Johnny was barely conscious, and Henry's bleeding had mostly stopped. Algot and I secured the horses as best we could while others came to help. I don't remember much about the rest of the morning, except that I was relegated to the farmhouse and threshing was ended for the day.

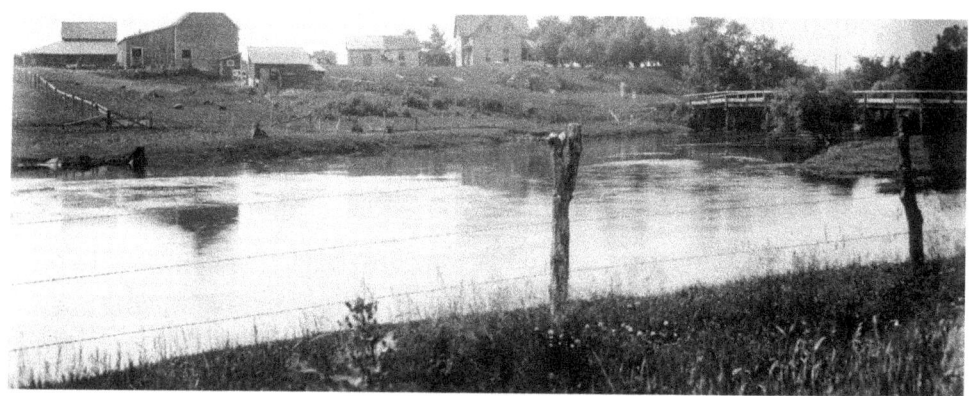

View from the field of the runaway looking back at the Groundhouse River and the farmstead, circa 1930

IMMIGRANT FARMS

The next day threshing was resumed with borrowed wagons and new neighbor volunteers. Henry had his face stitched up in Mora, and Johnny stayed a few days in the hospital with a concussion. He subsequently lost his farm, maybe in part due to the residual effects of his fall and resultant brain injury. In the weeks to come, Grandpa gave me lessons in posthole digging and in stretching barbed wire to repair the damaged fence. The next year most of the neighbors had replaced their horses with small Ford Ferguson tractors.

Sixty years later while I was helping my mother to tend the family grave sites in the Brunswick Lutheran Church cemetery, I asked how her grandfather Molin, my great-grandfather, died in 1916. "Oh, he fell off a hayrack in a runaway and died a few days later."

I have many other farm stories, but should tell you about butchering. Each December one of the pigs was kept from market for use on the farm. The four other pigs were sold along with eggs for cash income.

One winter I wanted to be there when they slaughtered the Christmas pig. It was arranged for a Saturday morning, so that I could be present. I must have been about twelve. My father and I were hunters, and I was used to dressing pheasants, ducks, and grouse. But I had never seen a large animal butchered.

After school on a Friday, I took the Greyhound bus to Brunswick to witness the next day's ritual. I had experienced how much of the pig was used at the farm table. Roasts and chops were common on Sundays. Dad relished pig knuckles and salt pork. Headcheese and blood cake were Christmas delicacies enjoyed by the initiated.

Saturday morning arrived. The milking and other chores in the barn were completed, a full meat-eggs-and-potato breakfast was eaten, and we headed to the pig barn for the lone remaining hog. Julius Sundboom, the local, untrained, self-taught veterinarian, had been hired to lead the butchering team. Grandmother gave me a large metal pan to catch the blood. Grandpa stayed busy in the barn until the event was over. It was then I realized why Grandma was the one who taught me how to kill and clean chickens.

When we entered the hog barn, Julius asked if I could handle a gun. When I said yes, he handed me a light rifle, gave instructions on where to shoot the pig, how he would cut the neck, and where I was to catch the blood in my pan.

"Are you ready?"

"I guess so."

"OK. Shoot!"

I shot the pig between the eyes, Julius flashed a knife to the staggering pig's neck, and I brought my pan to catch the pulsating blood. The deep pan was almost full as the animal was laid back and the blood stopped flowing.

As I left the hog barn, I carried the steaming pan in the cold December air across the snowy yard to the house. Grandma was waiting and ready to make what she called "blud kaka," which translates to "blood cake." This was a Christmas-breakfast tradition that I had learned to like, and now I understood its origin.

The next two days were spent cutting the meat, boiling the pig's head in a large copper kettle on the woodstove for headcheese, and stuffing sausage. Some of the meats were salted for preservation. The feet and knuckles were cooked and pickled. The meat and cartilage from the head were combined with gelatine to make what was known as "silta" (also called headcheese). All these delicacies would be added to lutefisk and Swedish meatballs for holiday meals. We still eat some of these foods during the Christmas holidays. Lutefisk has been replaced by halibut. So far no substitute has been found for blood cake.

In 1951 I was fourteen when my grandparents traded the farm for a resort near Nisswa, Minnesota. Their farm was becoming difficult for them to manage. Two of Grandmother's brothers lived in nearby Brainerd, so it was a good move that lasted nearly ten years.

IMMIGRANT FARMS

I look back fondly on the days I spent in Brunswick. They were a major complement to the urban life we had in Minneapolis. I had a good idea of how crops were planted and harvested and how farm animals were raised and came to the table. There wasn't much I didn't know about animal procreation, which made any parental birds-and-bees talk superfluous.

I didn't realize it at the time, but the tight-knit Swedish-immigrant community was changing. Most of the sons and daughters of my age left the community or worked in local towns. Their farms gradually became a hobby or second occupation. The Swedish Lutheran church has successfully transitioned to an ecumenical religious community-gathering place and maintains its cemetery. The Swedish Baptist church has dissolved and now houses the town hall. The creamery, feed store, and co-op store have closed. Many of the buildings are gone. The main highway now skirts the old town center.

I still go to Brunswick each spring to tend the family graves. Four great-grandparents, four grandparents, my parents, several aunts, an uncle, and cousins are buried there. As I kneel to cut away encroaching grass, clean the markers, and plant new flowers, I reminisce about each individual who was part of my life and how they helped develop the person I am today.

My experiences on the Hanson and Larson farms have left other impressions. I still like to grow things and keep a vegetable garden every summer. I'm not very good with flowers and only keep what I call a "very wild flower garden."

When my wife Gail and I considered a site for a vacation home, we started with an undeveloped eighty-acre tract of wooded land. We built a log cabin, a log garage, and created some trails. Poplar trees from the property were milled for flooring, and birch logs were turned into cabinets. Our own large pines were spared, but we helped cut, haul, and peel the red pine logs we used from our builder's land a few miles away.

DO NO HARM

My first outside purchase was a 1952 Ferguson tractor, including a back blade, scoop, and five-foot cutter to attach to the three-point lift. So far we haven't sheeted the outside of our buildings with siding or plastered the inside walls. The new Hanson land supports no domestic animals, but the garden supplies summer vegetables and berries. It's not a working farm, but as I grade the road or work in the woods with my tractor, i am reminded of my youth and the family farms in Brunswick.

CHAPTER SIX

Canoes, Camps, and Cabins

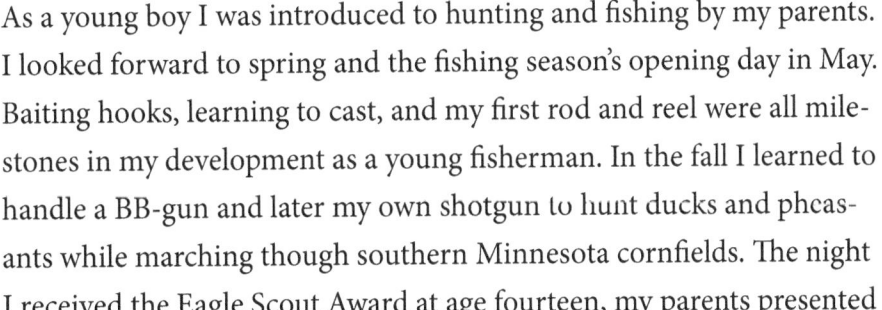

As a young boy I was introduced to hunting and fishing by my parents. I looked forward to spring and the fishing season's opening day in May. Baiting hooks, learning to cast, and my first rod and reel were all milestones in my development as a young fisherman. In the fall I learned to handle a BB-gun and later my own shotgun to hunt ducks and pheasants while marching though southern Minnesota cornfields. The night I received the Eagle Scout Award at age fourteen, my parents presented me with a 12-gauge, model 12 Winchester shotgun. I was destined for a lifelong pursuit of birds and fish.

During a Boy Scout canoe trip the summer of 1952 into the northern Minnesota and Canadian Boundary Waters Canoe Area (BWCA), I also became excited about canoes and camping. I was with a group of thirteen teenage boys with a college-student guide heading north from the Region Ten canoe base on Moose Lake near Ely, Minnesota. We spent 10 days learning the ways and skills of the fur-trading Voyageurs from 200 years ago. By the end of the trip we were running across portages with packs on our backs and a wood canoe on our shoulders. I was hooked.

My first three years at Dartmouth were confined to premed studies, basketball, and summer construction work in order to pay for the next year of college. At the time I couldn't engage in frivolous activities like fishing, hunting, and canoeing. However, I found more time for recreation in medical school. I would plan to spend Saturday noon to Sunday afternoon away from lectures and studying. I took up downhill and cross-country skiing in the winter and canoeing and fishing in the warmer months. The Mascoma River, a few miles south of Hanover, was a great white-water stream each spring. The Dartmouth College Land Grant near the Canada-New Hampshire border was much like the boundary waters in Minnesota. There were no large lakes, but the Swift and Dead Diamond rivers guided my canoe to wild fishing spots among pine trees, rocks, ledges, and waterfalls. I enjoyed sleeping in the open along the river and having trout for dinner and breakfast.

When I came back to Minnesota to finish medical school, John Kersey — a longtime friend from south Minneapolis who also attended Dartmouth Medical School — and I made several canoe trips.

We canoed one Saturday down the Wisconsin Brule River, which empties into Lake Superior's south shore. It was spring, the river was fast and high, and it was the opening day of steelhead fishing. We were having a great time, paddling hard at times to control our canoe, and shooting white-water rapids. The river was lined with fishermen. When we came to what looked like the biggest rapids of the day, we had just enough time to look at each other. John's look said, "Let's go for it."

As we steered to the deepest slot between two large rocks, we saw that the drop was more than we expected, more like a small falls. The bow of our canoe nosed into the rushing water below the falls, and the canoe rolled over and swamped us in the cold May water. The hole below the falls was deep so we had no footing. We wrestled our water-filled canoe to an eight-foot bank. We turned over the canoe to empty it. As I looked up, I saw a large man above us standing on the edge and watching us extricate ourselves and the canoe from the river. I noticed that he was holding a large trout by the gills near his waist. The fishtail was dragging on the ground. "Where did you get that fish?" I asked. Pointing to the deep water hole from which we had emerged, he said, "Oh, right about there."

We were two wet, cold, red-faced canoeists trying to apologize to a stoic, unsmiling fisherman for spoiling his fishing hole. But we had a story that has been told and relived many times through the years.

After Gail and I were married, we had little time to canoe and camp while raising two toddlers and moving to Japan for three years. Gail had made a camping trip in California once, and she had spent summer vacations at an uncle's resort in northern Minnesota before we were married. But she did not have much experience hunting or fishing.

On returning to Minnesota from Japan in 1968, I resumed my training program in internal medicine at the Minneapolis VA Hospital. As a hospital staff member, I was able to rent an apartment in the former bachelor-officer quarters on the old Fort Snelling grounds. On the opening day of duck season in October, John Kersey and I planned to go hunting on the Carlos Avery Game Reserve about forty miles north of the Twin Cities. Our three-year-old son, Peter, asked, "What is hunting ducks?" I tried to explain that I was going out to a waterway to shoot ducks with a gun. "Do you mean the ducks we watch at the lake?" When I said yes, he immediately said, "I want to go, too."

That day John and I went back to where we had hunted while in medical school three years earlier. The scene had changed. A dam had raised the water level so that what was then a marsh with a small stream was now almost a lake, crowded with coots (also called mudhens). As we approached every potential place to find cover, other hunters stood up. Finally we found a spot of dry land on which to pull up our canoe and stand, about fifteen minutes before the noon season opening. Then a slow-flying heron came into view and the first gunshot rang out. Any ducks in flight rose out of range, and the raft of coots moved about twenty feet and resettled in the open water.

The shooting continued at any out-of-range flying object without any hits that we could see. Finally, after about an hour and a half, we decided we had had enough. We climbed back into our canoe for a paddle down the wide, slow-moving Sunrise River to our car. A flock of coots rose up in front of us. "Bang, bang, bang," came shots from both shores passing about ten yards in front of us. We could feel the percussion and hear the pellets whiz just off our canoe's bow. Our first reaction was to duck. Then we yelled at the hunters to let us pass. When we finally reached our car and loaded the canoe on top, we headed to the Stacy Cafe in the closest town to settle our nerves. That was the last time either of us has gone hunting. I still have my Winchester Model 12 at our cabin, but it hasn't been fired in almost fifty years.

Other memorable canoe stories include the cigarettes, candy, and wine trip to the Boundary Waters Canoe Area in northern Minnesota while attending medical school. Or the multiple family trips we took on the Wisconsin Flambeau and Namakagon rivers. During one trip on the Namakagon our family of four and our gear were so soaked after a cold, rainy May day that I drove the two hours back to Minneapolis in my boxer shorts with the car heater on full.

We also took a car-tenting trip in the early 1970s that made us reconsider any future tent-camping vacations. We stopped at a nice state-park campground just over the Idaho-Oregon border at the end of a long day driving west. It was a wide-open area on a hillside sloping toward the Snake River. There were few other campers, so we had our choice of campsites. As the four of us put up our tent and began cooking a meal, a gentle breeze began to get stronger as the sun was setting. By the time we were ready to eat, there were serious gusts of wind. We sat at a picnic table next to our tent spooning noodle soup into our mouths. A gust of wind blew my noodles off the spoon into daughter

Marta's face and lap. We started to laugh when the same thing happened to Gail, who was sitting at the end of the table so the broth and noodles hit the ground. Just then, the tent blew down and collapsed onto the table and our meal. We couldn't set the tent back up, and our meal was mostly on the ground. When I talked to the park ranger about what we might expect for the rest of the night, he said, "See those trees over there?" Across the barren hillside were two scrawny, stunted trees bent in the direction of the wind. "Those trees are permanently bent. When the wind starts, it usually lasts for two or three days." A truckers' motel became our refuge for the night.

We enjoyed camping but decided that getting off the ground was a good idea. We bought a small pop-up trailer the next year and traveled to eastern Canada and the maritime provinces including the Gaspe Peninsula. We had also begun going to Camp du Nord, a YMCA family camp on the edge of the BWCA. There were age-appropriate group activities in the morning and swimming and canoeing in the afternoons. Most years we took an overnight canoe trip into the BWCA. Hook Lake was our favorite destination.

Hook Lake was at the end of a three-lake, three-portage paddle that took half a day. The fishing was usually good, but we brought other supplies just in case. One year the four of us were fishing from the canoe after an evening meal. We had some fish on a stringer when Marta said she had a bite. Her pole action suggested she might be right. As we watched her reeling in what seemed like a modest fish or a large weed, her pole bent further, and she began struggling to make any headway in retrieving the line. When she finally brought her catch near the boat, we saw a small fish on her line that was in the mouth of a large northern pike. We didn't have a net and the light line was no match for the monster fish. The big fish dove down and the line broke. We did have fish on our stringer, but the fish we called Walter from the movie *On Golden Pond* would live to excite future campers. That could have been the end of the story. When we arrived at our campsite, it was getting dark, and we decided to clean our fish in the morning and left them in the water. That night the turtles had a feast. All that remained in the morning were fish heads still attached to our stringer.

Camp du Nord became our family's cabin in the woods for a week in the summer and long weekends in the fall and winter. Both Gail and I had fond memories of going "up North" to cabins with our families. Camp du Nord filled that recreational need for us and freed us from ownership and maintenance, allowing us to travel to other interesting places in the world.

This arrangement served us well during the 1970s and 1980s. Then in 1991 Gail's siblings began talking about their experiences at a fishing resort near Bemidji, Minnesota, run by their aunt and uncle. The resort had been repurchased by their cousins and had been significantly modernized. "Why don't we have our own family cabin?" was her brothers' cry. We spent the spring searching for a place in northern Minnesota and western Wisconsin. We found a property on Lake Namakagon near Cable, Wisconsin. The property was twice the distance from the Twin Cities than we had wished, it cost twice as much as we had budgeted for, and it was half as big as desired. On the plus side it was a log building and it came with a stone fireplace and a beach.

As it worked out, we had six families to share a two-bedroom, one living-dining-kitchen-room cabin. We winterized the cabin with an insulating roof, we converted a tool shed to a bunkhouse, and added a screen porch. One out of six weeks it was ours to use — an arrangement that worked surprisingly well for over a decade even as the participants moved and changed lifestyles and interests.

For years Gail and I had avoided owning a second property. We preferred to choose varied vacation travel around the United States and abroad, since we did not want to be tied down to one location. But as

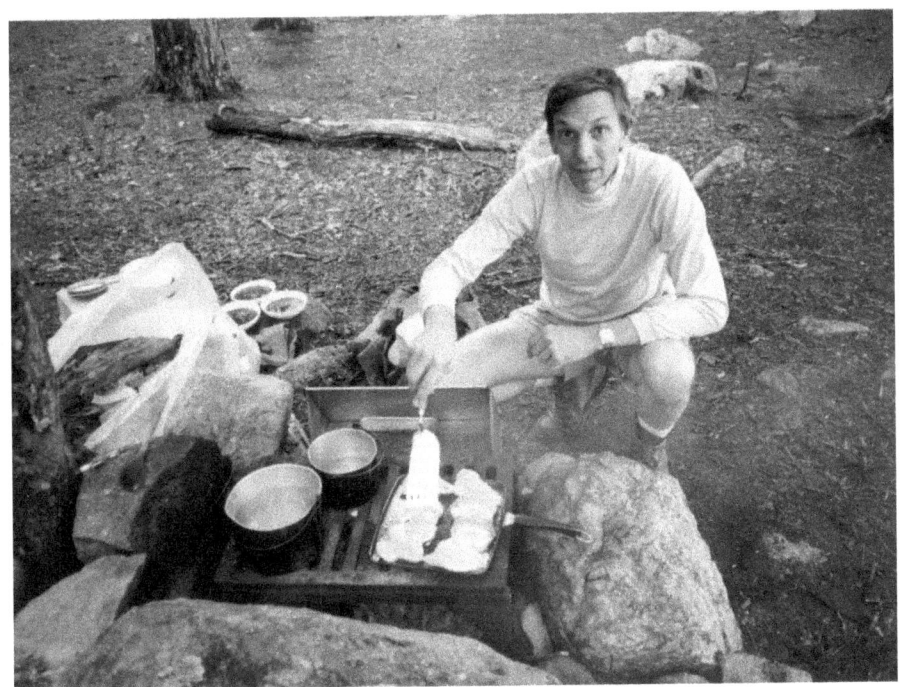

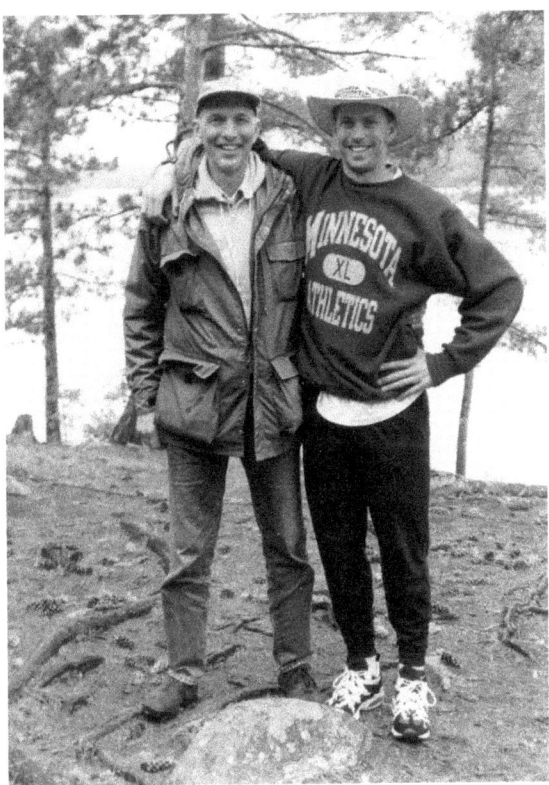

Canoeing and camping, 1970s and 1980s

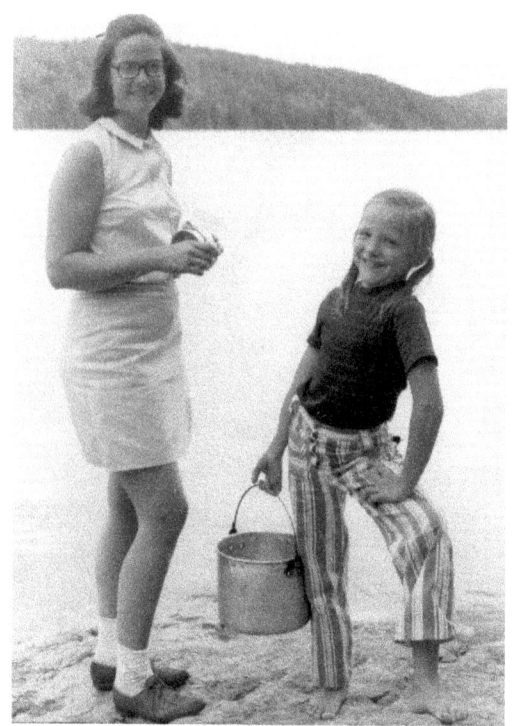
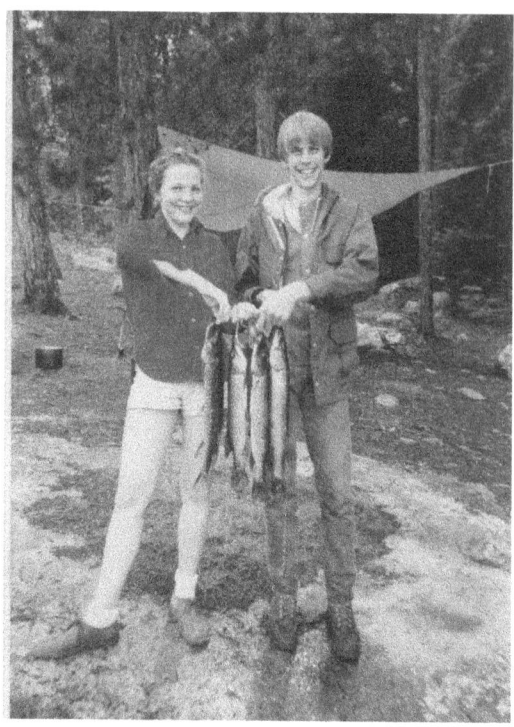
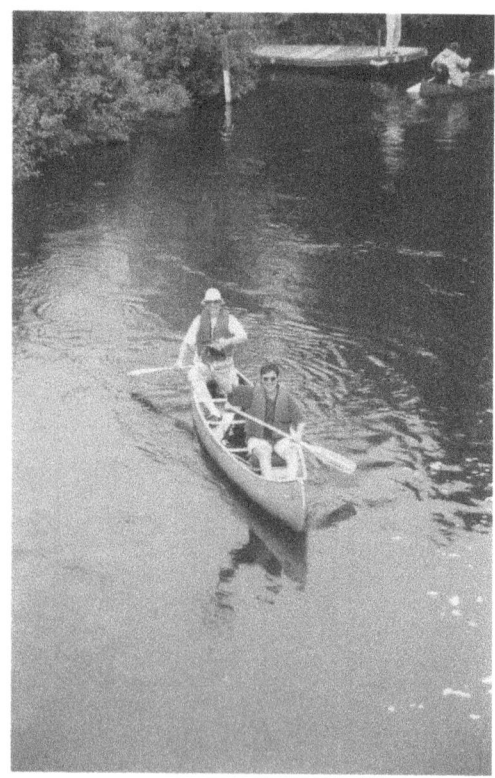

Canoeing and camping, 1970s and 1980s

we acclimated to our weeks on Lake Namakagon, we began to reconsider. Perhaps we could find a lake lot for future options.

During the fall of 1993 we had several interesting opportunities. An 80-acre parcel encompassing a channel between the 200-acre Jackson Lake and the nearly 3,000-acre Lake Namakagon was listed. I was unable to find the borders of the property. The realtor had sent other prospects out to look, but they couldn't even locate the property. A plot map showed that the property covered both sides of a marshy channel, had wide access to Jackson Lake, and contained fifty acres of woods. I decided to pace out what I thought might be the property borders on high ground. I walked on a compass-line a quarter mile west and a quarter mile south, then tried to find my way back to the overgrown access road. The channel and marsh borders were less accessible by land, but could be accessed from the water. We made an offer to the owner, a hunter who lived in southern Wisconsin. Our offer was just over half the asking price and we requested a survey. His counter offer didn't reduce the price much and eliminated the survey. That stopped the negotiations. Thinking we had lost our chance at the property, we returned to our lives back in Minneapolis.

Snow came in mid-November that year. The family's cabin on Lake Namakagon was snug and warm. We were making plans to do some cross-country skiing after Thanksgiving when we received a call from the Realtor. "Are you still interested in the property you saw last fall?" My response was, "Yes, but you told us we were not in the seller's ballpark on price." "Well, the seller is anxious to sell. He told me not to lose that buyer." I told Gail, "I think we need to go back and ski the line."

This time it didn't take long to make a deal. We gave up on the survey and slightly raised our offer. We started to think about building a cabin on this most unusual property containing water, marsh, and woods of mature oak, birch, aspen, maple, and pine. I discovered that it held eleven of the sixteen habitats of the Great North Woods — it had most of the natural environments we enjoyed from canoeing and camping trips. We were going to build a cabin. Sometime.

At that time a close friend became ill. A member of our wedding party was dying, and she wanted to go to the Amazon as one of her last wishes. We went with her. When we came home, we looked at each other and said, "If we want a cabin of our own, we should do it now while we can." So began a two-year project to build first a log garage and then a log cabin. Soon we called it "Cabin Two (or C-2)" as opposed to "Cabin One (C-1)," our shared family cabin which is down our channel on Lake Namakagon.

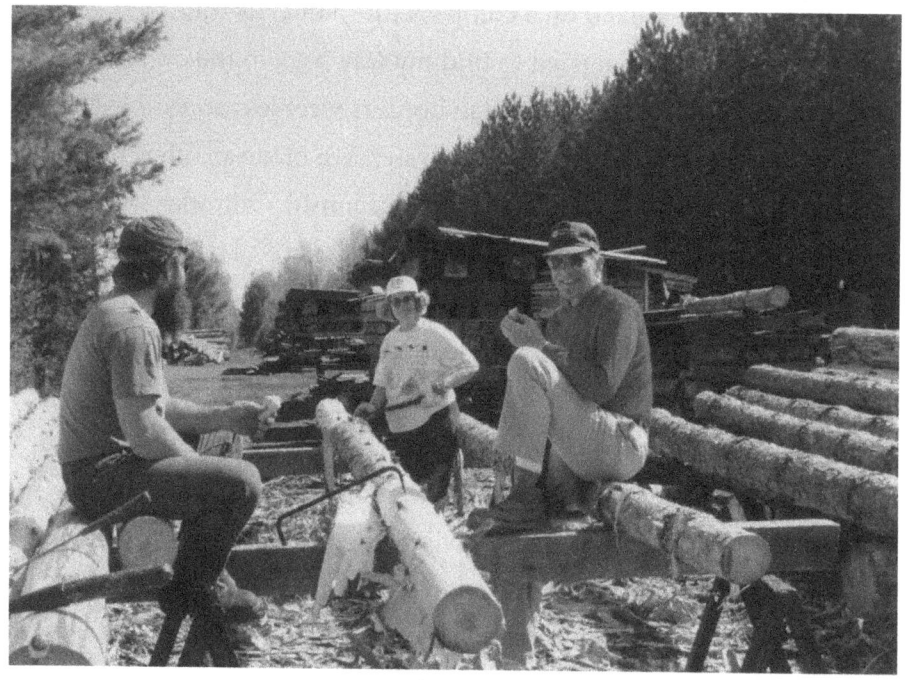

Peeling cabin logs with Dan Dums our builder, 1996

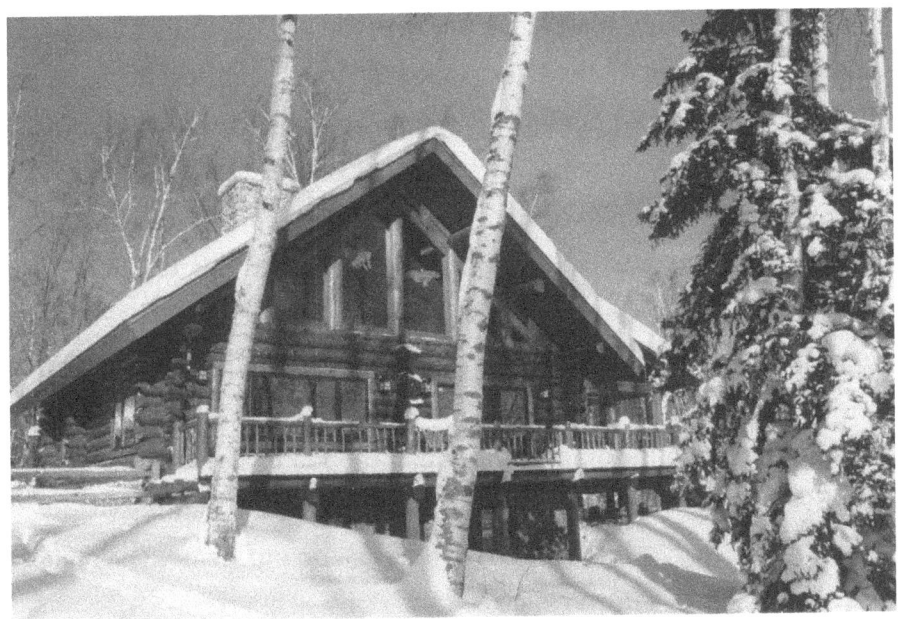

The Jackson Lake cabin

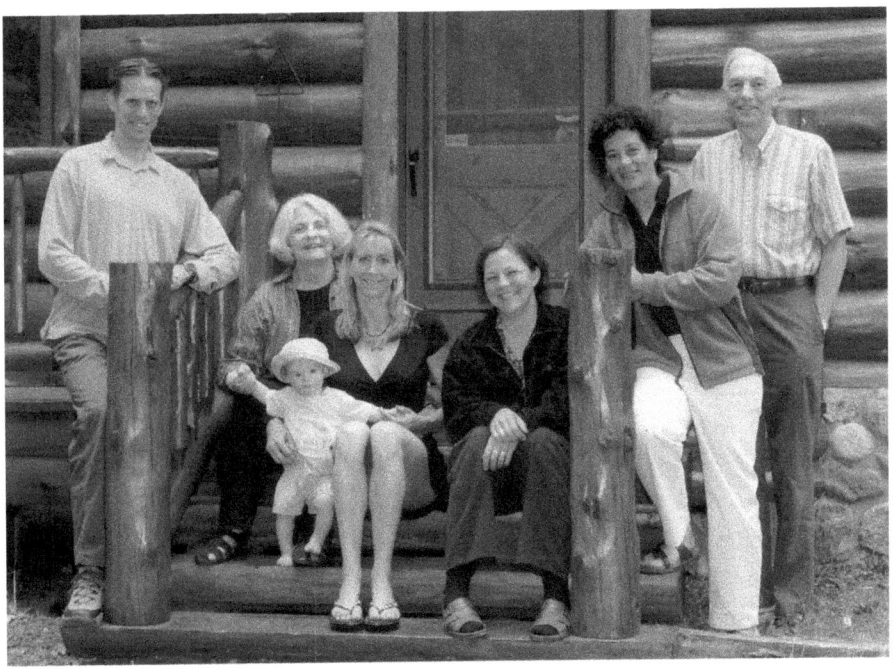

Family summer of 2008. Left to right: Peter, Gail, Halen (six months), Elise Fett (Halen's mother), Marta, Kelly, and me

DO NO HARM

It has been twenty years since we finished C-2. We easily traded canoes and sleeping on the ground for year-round comfort during our nature rejuvenations. I have a 1952 Ferguson tractor made in Canada that is similar to Grandfather Larson's 1948 Ford made in the United States. We have ski trails to maintain, birds to watch, a private road to grade, a garden to tend, and firewood to collect and split. Gail has a design and quilting space. In our gravel driveway turtles lay their eggs, which animals dig up and eat at night. Birds, bears, deer, and wolves pass by. Friends and family visit off and on, but mostly it's just the two of us enjoying the quiet at the end of the road. We read, quilt, eat simply, and enjoy time in the woods. It connects us to nature's yearly cycles, the animals, plants, and trees that sustain our living. The night sky connects us to a universe far beyond our reach.

CHAPTER SEVEN

Championship Seasons

"Sports will make a man out of you."

"Being part of a sports team will teach you lessons
you will use the rest of your life."

These were the statements from some of our coaches as they taught us the skills of football, basketball, and baseball. Most of us were just anxious to play. The dedication of men such as Jack Marton, Don Sovell, Bob Ottness, and Warren Ajax teaching football, basketball, and baseball skills to groups of eager junior-high-school boys paid off in city and state championships a few years later.

By the time I reached high school I had been designated as an end in football, a forward in basketball, and a first baseman in baseball. Our youth coaches turned us over to high-school teachers who were often coaching to supplement their incomes. Ray Smith coached football. He often had excellent high-school athletes, but had never won a championship. His American history classes were ponderous, soporific, and boring. Football practice wasn't much better, but at least we were outside. In retrospect, he was not inspiring, and our junior-year record in the fall of 1953 was mediocre.

Coming into our senior year, our team was determined to do better. When we started practice in August, we were surprised to find a new coach. Marv Helling had been hired to replace Coach Smith. He quickly made it clear that he was in charge and had high expectations. He was not planning to build a new team for the future; he was going to make us champions now.

After a week of practice, he took many of us aside and explained what he expected from each of us and what we needed to work on. Coach Helling had a bright but serious smile. Within a few days we knew there was a new man in charge.

By the time the league preview was held on the first Friday night of the school year, the team had a new attitude, new fundamental skills, and an inspiring leader. Each team in the league played for a quarter that night. This was our first chance to see the other ten teams. (One team played two quarters to round out the six-quarter event.)

The first full game with North High School was said to be the toughest game of the season. Their quarterback could be the league's best. I made some tackles in the first quarter. The next thing I remember was lining up for a play at the end of the third quarter. As I settled into a three-point offensive stance, a referee blew his whistle, picked up the ball, and moved to the other end of the field. I chased after him asking what was happening? What penalty had we incurred?

He quickly recognized I was confused and needed to be removed from the game. A physician checked me out, and when I tried reentering the game my helmet was nowhere to be found. Mike Olson, our student manager, said the coach told him not to let me have it. I was out of the game. I had played the second and third quarters, attended a halftime talk, yet had no recollection of anything.

CHAMPIONSHIP SEASONS

This was decades before concussion protocols and brain scans. A cursory physician's exam wisely kept me out of that game, which we won. I rode the bus back to school where my parents picked me up. I slept poorly, and the next morning l awoke with a splitting headache. I had had a major concussion, but by Monday I went back to school. I joined football practice and prepared for the next game without further medical evaluation.

The next week I participated in activities as though I was fine. On Friday another game was played on our home field. I played the first half and thought I was doing well. We were easily winning, but on an offensive drive near the end of the second quarter, I missed a block and caught my leg in a tangle. Not realizing that I had broken my right fibula, I walked back to the huddle. On the next play a pass to me was called near the goal line. I went out five yards, turned to my left, and Clyde Smith placed the ball in my hands for a touchdown. As l limped off the field, an assistant coach asked if I was OK. A substitute was sent in. That was the last time I played a football game. The small fibula bone in my right leg was shattered, the next week I was fitted with a long-leg walking cast that broke while I was playing pickup touch football. The doctor then fixed me with a short-leg cast that required four weeks using crutches.

I was fortunate to play with a group of good athletes who came together as a team under a new coach. Our team was the undefeated winner of the city championship during the regular season. Our star running back, Jon Spolum, dislocated his shoulder in the final league game. He and I walked the sidelines as the team came up short in a postseason game with Central High School, the St. Paul city champion. The season was over before my leg recovered. Years later, I wondered if the missed block and broken leg were related to my concussion the week before.

Basketball season started within weeks of the end of the football season. Several of us were now turning our attention to another sport requiring different skills. My right leg had withered in the cast. I had no physical therapy, not even a consultation with a trainer. Getting back in shape for basketball was up to me.

At practice it was clear I had a long way to go. The previous year I was a starter — now I was limping and not competitive. I questioned whether I would recover in time to make the team. Our team expected us to do well. A loss in our second December preseason game led to a team meeting that included some former players. Complaints about our aging coach, Ray Ross, were aired. He made us shoot underhand free throws and taught a two-handed, standing set shot. He didn't like us to shoot jump shots. At the meeting the former players said it was up to us to to make our season with the coach we had. We had had a winning football season; now it was up to us to do the same in basketball.

Some changes were coming. I was recovering from my withered leg. Our longtime center, who was six foot two and had begun shaving in seventh grade was now the same height as a high-school senior. Gordie Sundin was our tallest player at six five, but he was best at forward. Lee Chapman, good at shooting and driving, and Pat Sweeney, a ball handler, were the best guards. The year preceding we had convinced our coach, who had a 1930s view of how basketball should be played, that David Michaelson could play forward, and I could be designated center. He accepted our suggestions. In reality we played with two guards and three forwards that season. David Wiggins, Jack Medcalf, Neil Feinberg, and Tal Tischer were our senior reserves.

By January, when the Minneapolis high-school basketball season began, we had established a starting lineup and we started to win games. As our offense developed and our defense improved, our confidence grew. We won all our conference games and the city championship. Now we were faced with postseason play — one loss and the season would be over.

Minnesota had one boys' state basketball tournament in 1955. Eight

CHAMPIONSHIP SEASONS

regional teams played off over three days. We knew the competition in our region would be tough. A suburban team, St. Louis Park, had recruited one of the best city players to join a team that had played well the year before. We had scrimmaged with them during the regular season and we knew their strengths. We didn't know of any weaknesses.

But before we could play in the regional tournament, we had to win our district. We were playing teams we had played during the regular season. We tried to take games as they came and not look ahead, but we knew St. Louis Park was the strongest team in our way to reaching the state tournament.

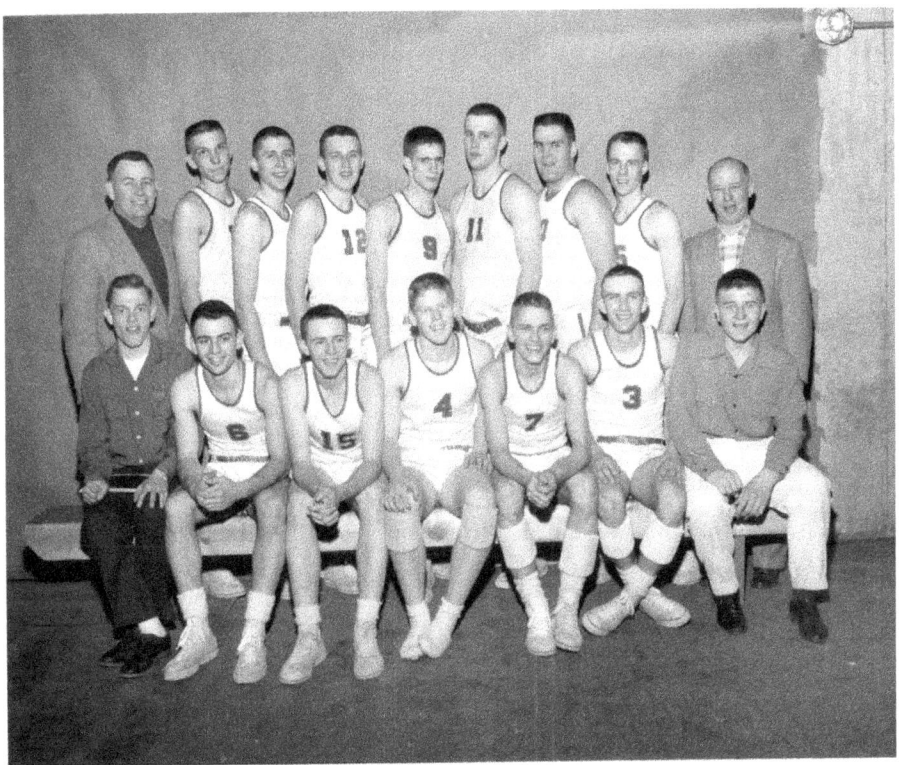

Washburn High School State Tournament Team, 1955
First row: Lindholm (junior manager), Feinberg, Murphy, Chapman, Wiggins, Sweeney, Olson (senior manager)
Second row: Helleckson (assistant coach), me, Hedin, Knudtson, Michaelson, Sundin, Tischer, Medcalf, Ross (coach)

We won our district and the first regional games. As predicted, the St. Louis Park team met us in the regional finals. It was a tough game for us, but we played well and won. Washburn was in the state tournament for the third time in twenty-five years. Two teams in the 1940s had failed to reach the finals under Coach Ross, but this was 1955, and the game had changed. We didn't know what to expect from the Greater Minnesota teams. New Prague, a farming community south of the Twin Cities, had a highly touted center, and Austin had what they called their "twin-towers" centers. These players were all six foot six or taller. We didn't have a comparable center. I was only six three.

We played the first game of the eight-team tournament on a Thursday afternoon in March. Morris is a medium-sized state-university town in western Minnesota. They had a good outside shooter. Their center was supposed to be the heart of the team — and my defensive assignment. I was nervous warming up. We were playing on the University of Minnesota's raised court in front of 15,000 spectators.

After several times up and down the court, I realized that although their center was big, he was slow. He couldn't defend a drive to the basket, and he could be boxed out for rebounds. His supporting players were handled easily by the rest of our team. By halftime we had a commanding lead, and our reserves finished the game.

The winner of the next game would be our opponent the following night. We watched as the tall, agile, athletic center from New Prague, Ron Johnson, dominated the game. This team would clearly give us more competition. We watched as their soft passes were repeatedly lobbed to him for easy layups. It became clear we had to keep the ball away from him if we were going to have a chance. We also noticed that the guards and forwards were rarely shooting from the outside, often missed when they did shoot, and relied on Johnson to get the rebound.

Coach Ross asked us how we thought we should defend against this intimidating center. Gordie Sundin, at six five, was our tallest player and was the obvious choice to guard behind him. I thought we should sag in front of him in a double team, thus making it difficult for him to get the ball. Also it would be important to box him out from rebounds, which seemed to be a big part of his game.

The game went well the next night. We squeezed Johnson with our double-team defense, muscled him away from rebounds, and let their guards shoot and miss. The plan worked. We won with some ease. I scored twenty-nine points, my highest total in high school.

The arena held about 18,000 spectators for the championship game with Austin on Saturday evening. Austin was a frequent participant in state tournaments. It is the home of Spam and Hormel Foods, which supports and invests in high-school athletics with considerable success. Their "twin-tower" centers would be a challenge. Their outside shooters were good. We couldn't afford double teams on two big centers. Gordie and I had to match up with them one-on-one.

The score was close early in the game until one of our players got into foul trouble. Our first substitute and sixth man, David Wiggins, came into the game. He was a guard-forward who had been an effective replacement of anyone who was in foul trouble or having an off night. As soon as he entered the game he intercepted a pass, drove toward the basket, and scored. He defended their best outside player, made drives and passes that led to a lead we never gave up. It looked to others as if we coasted to a win, but on the floor I was exhausted and was glad when the buzzer sounded. The postgame celebration went on around several of us who were glad to find the bench and rest. At the awards ceremony, Sundin, Sweeney, and I were named to the all-state tournament team.

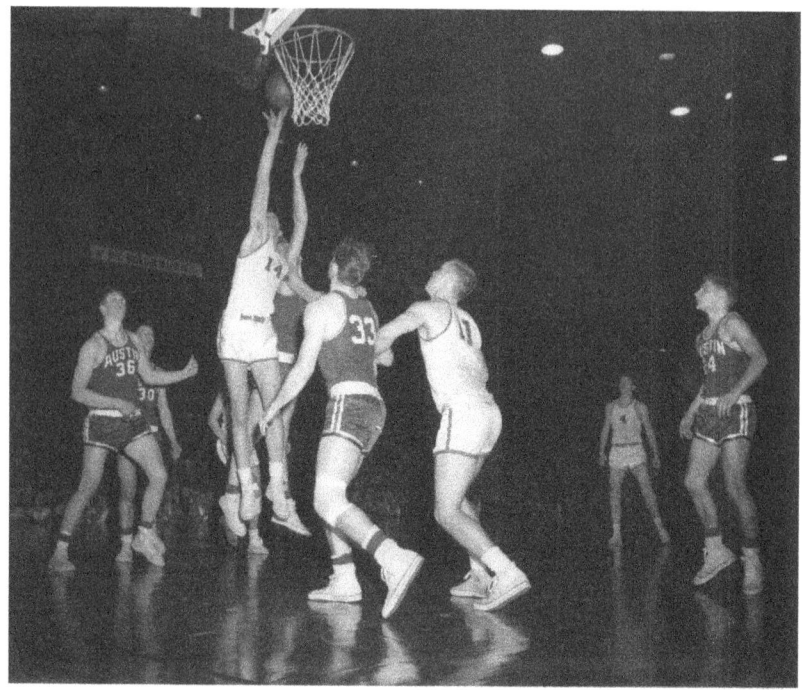

Chamionship game, Washburn vs Austin
Chapman #4, Sundin #11, me #14

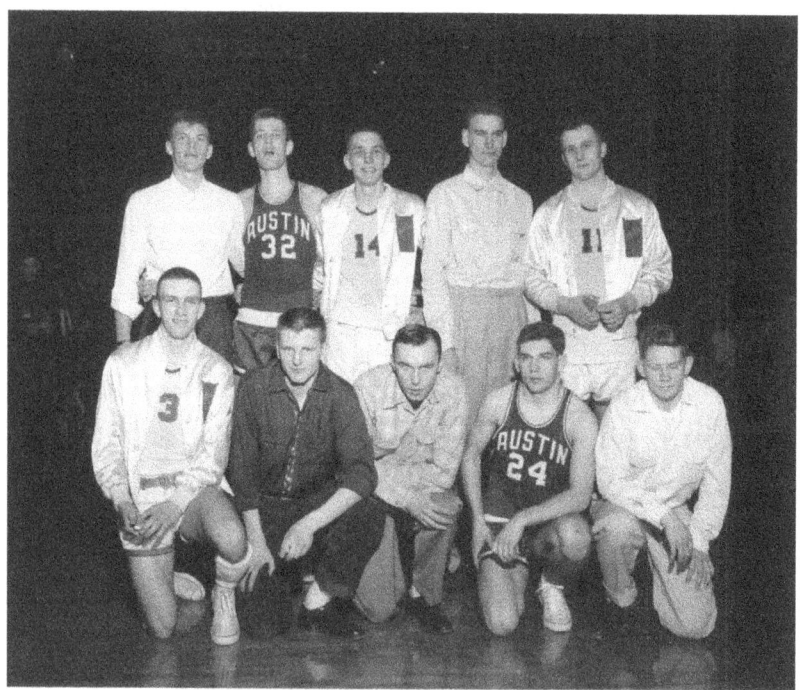

All-State Tournament Team. Pat Sweeney #3, Gordie Sundin #11.
I am in the middle of the back row. Ron Johnson from New Prague is on
my left and Jerry Olson (one of Austin's twin towers) is on my right.

Our senior class was feeling good after winning major athletic championships in both football and basketball. The swimming, golf, and tennis teams were to receive city recognition. Baseball started in April, and Coach Ross had us getting ready for a short season as soon as the fields dried. For many players, we had one more season before graduating in June.

I was tall but slow and weak. At first base I could stop most balls thrown or hit. At bat I could make contact, but the hits didn't go very far. Gordie Sundin was an intimidating pitcher and rightfielder. Jon Spolum, the running back who dislocated his shoulder, was our strongest pitcher and centerfielder. David Wiggins, the basketball energizer, played shortstop. Pat Sweeney, our place kicker in football and basketball guard, was our third baseman. Tom Dubay and Bob Reitow pitched. Three juniors: Ed Munson (catcher), Bruce Sachs (second base), and John Councilman (outfield) completed the starting team.

The season progressed much as basketball had. We won all the regular season games. When the postseason district tournament started, we were experienced and knew what to expect. We had a strong pitching staff and position players who could catch and hit. We kept winning. We won both district and regional tournaments and were in another eight-team state tournament. Then came our June graduation, the evening before we were to play our first game ninety miles away in Rochester, Minnesota. The night of the dance and all-night graduation party we had to head home at 10:00 p.m. to face a restless night before another big game.

The International Falls team was our first obstacle. Their first baseman was the son of a famous Minnesota athlete, Bronco Nagerski. I was walked three times and was hit once in my four plate appearances. It turned out to be an easy win as was the game the following night. Now we were in another state-championship game — Austin was once again our opponent.

Austin had two good pitchers. Gary Underhill was its best and he pitched left-handed. As a right-handed hitter, I loved lefties. We won another state title. When the awards were given, I was surprised to be selected as first baseman on the all-state tournament team. Most of my production had been walks, being hit as a batter, and fielding low throws from our infielders.

That was a special year for Washburn High School athletics. The class of 1955, which met first in junior high as seventh graders, had brought athletic success to the school. Most of us attended college, and some became professors, engineers, dentists, physicians, military officers, bankers, and businessmen. Pat Sweeney, the place kicker in football, guard in basketball, and baseball third baseman had a multisport career in college and became a security expert. Lee Chapman, the basketball guard, played at the University of Minnesota before becoming an orthodontist. David Michaelson played basketball at the University of Colorado before becoming successful in business. Gordie Sundin signed a major league baseball contract with Baltimore and played seven years before entering a business career. Jon Spolum, the power running back and baseball pitcher, played football for the University of Colorado and minor league baseball in Wisconsin before he became a successful salesman in men's clothing. I went on to play basketball at Dartmouth College and became a pulmonary-and-critical-care-medicine physician.

Sixty years later it is hard to believe the success we had in our highschool years. We had some exceptional players, but no dominating star. In order to succeed, we had to play as a team, which made all the difference. Teamwork, cooperation, respect for others, discipline, tolerance, fairness, and caring for one another were attributes we gained and carried to the activities that have defined our lives since.

I cannot say I have an intimate understanding of high-school athletics today. Our grandson is starting to play individual and team sports at a younger age than I did. It seems young athletes are encouraged to focus more on one, or at most two sports, at an earlier age, to the point of playing one sport all year around. I enjoyed the three sports I played at the high-school level and developed a variety of friendships and skills that have ever since served me well.

Becoming an Adult

CHAPTER EIGHT

Athletics and Academics

What to do after high school? Sociologists have called this the first adult transition. I was considering a career as a physician, but the where and how were unclear. In junior-high school I was told that Latin and German languages would be required, but by the time I was seriously choosing courses in high school, those requirements were gone. I wanted to continue playing sports, if possible, and to attend a good academic institution that offered premed courses. I also had the idea that I should go far enough away from home so that I could not drop off my laundry on the weekends.

As I looked into various options, I was intrigued by the educational opportunities and the athletic philosophy of Ivy League schools. (This was before West-Coast schools like Stanford and UCLA were as highly regarded in the Midwest.) When I discussed my choice to apply to Harvard and Dartmouth, Miss Christensen, our school counselor, encouraged me to apply to a "backup school" in Minnesota. She was worried about my chances at acceptance, but both Dartmouth and Harvard had accepted Washburn graduates in previous years.

When acceptance letters arrived in April, I received two with enough financial aid from both schools to make them affordable. Now I had to make a decision between an urban university in Boston or a rural college in New Hampshire, neither of which I would visit before matriculating in September 1955. Both had sports teams in the division-one Ivy League, although neither had had much recent success. I was leaning toward Dartmouth because of its country location since I had grown up in a city.

Near the end of May I was invited to a Saturday lunch at the Minneapolis Athletic Club by the University of Minnesota basketball coach, Ossie Cowles. Several other students were there. I was seated with Coach Cowles and his assistant, Joe Vansisin. Cowles had lots of questions about what I wanted to do in college and after. Several of his current players had come from Minneapolis, so he was aware of the level of play. He asked about where I had applied to college and then why not Minnesota? As we finished our meal, he said, "I think you should go to Dartmouth." Later I found out he had coached Dartmouth to a national championship fifteen years earlier.

I decided not to play football at Dartmouth freshman year since I had had a concussion and a broken leg as a high-school senior. At least twenty-five freshmen turned out for basketball in the fall of 1955. We were surprised to be coached by Al Maguire, who had just retired from the National Basketball Association (NBA) and the New York Knickerbockers. After Dartmouth, Maguire went on to become an elite coach winning a national championship at Marquette University in 1977. He became a revered color commentator for men's college basketball during the NCAA's "March Madness" for years thereafter until he died of leukemia at age seventy-two.

Freshmen were not allowed to play varsity-team sports, but we had a fifteen-game freshman season across New England and New York. About the middle of the season Coach Maguire took Rudy Laruso

ATHLETICS AND ACADEMICS

and me aside onto the wooden bleachers away from the practicing team. Rudy was six foot seven and our center. Maguire said, "Laruso, you are big and our center, but you would fit best as a big forward in the NBA. You need to work on rebounding, making fifteen-foot jump shots, and driving to the basket from the corners." Rudy nodded and said, "Yes, Coach."

Then Coach turned to me. "Hanson, you will be a small forward or a shooting guard in the NBA. You need to work on ball handling, passing, driving, and shooting from the outside." He looked at me for a response. After a long pause while I collected my thoughts, I said, "I have never considered trying to play basketball beyond college as a career." "Well, you would play, if you could make it, wouldn't you?" he asked. When I gave a negative response, he was taken back. "I can't believe you wouldn't take a shot at it, if you could."

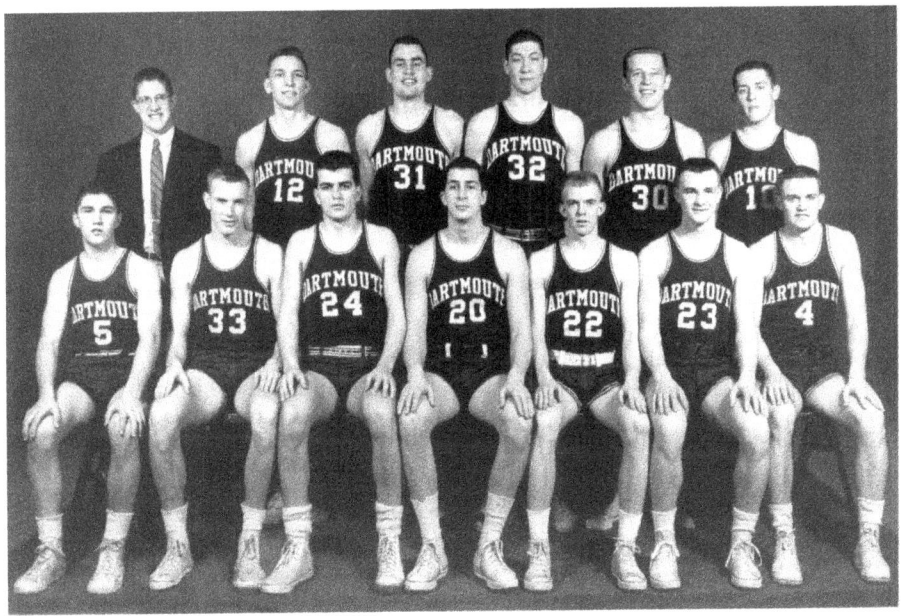

Dartmouth Freshman Basketball Team, 1955–56
Front row: Nick Porcinno, Tom Alley, Ed Hobbie,
Mickey Cohen, Bob Kline, Don DeVoe, "Rocky" Nelsen
Back row: Ted Harris (manager), me, Scott Palmer,
Rudy LaRusso, Rupert Schneider, Stan Drazen
Photograph copyright Dartmouth College. Printed with permission.

I think he felt all his players had visions of professional stardom, and I was not one of the boys. For the rest of the season, he called me "Doc" and asked me medical questions about diet, what to eat before games, and what to do about the strains and pains of my teammates.

Our freshman team did well. We played solid games and challenged the varsity in scrimmages. I don't remember losing any freshman games. The varsity won the Ivy League, but lost in the first round of the NCAA Tournament to West Virginia. Doggie Julian, a former Boston Celtics coach, led the varsity.

As a sophomore I was a bench rider, rarely playing with the game on the line. Coach Julian was a character. He had ideas about playing the game that we all absorbed. But his ideas about training, and especially about eating on game days, were subjects for humor books. We could not have mayonnaise on our dry turkey sandwiches. Salt was OK, but no butter. Only one glass of water. No carbonated or caffeinated beverages. We were hungry and thirsty with dry mouths by game time. We came in second to Yale and did not get into the NCAA postseason. Up to that point, athletics and academics had not clashed in my life, but that was about to change.

I practiced hard the summer of 1957 at home. After working all day as a plaster-tender (hod-carrier was the term used), I would go to the University of Minnesota field house to work out with university players. By Thanksgiving time I was on Dartmouth's starting lineup. But I needed to come late or miss practices due to afternoon labs in biochemistry. My lack of preparation must have shown, and by December I was back on the bench at the start of games. In January I was accepted to Dartmouth Medical School for the following school year beginning in September. Dartmouth offered entrance to the first two years of medical school after three undergraduate years.

The team did well, and I was an early substitute in most games. We won the Ivy-League championship and started a NCAA-tournament run. The Ivy-League winner was seeded in the 32-team tournament. The great Wilt Chamberlain, playing for Kansas, took up most of the basketball news that year. Ivy-League teams were expected to be finished after one game, but this year would be different.

We played our first game against the University of Connecticut in New York's Madison Square Garden. When we won, we advanced to the round of sixteen, which is now called the "Sweet Sixteen." We were to play the next weekend in Charlotte, North Carolina. For me, organic-chemistry labs were taking a toll. I had one foot in a winning basketball team and the other in a challenging chemistry course. Trying to learn chemistry on buses and planes wasn't working. I was getting more behind as the season's final weeks played out in March of 1958.

Our team packed up for the quarter-final weekend to be held in Charlotte at their new Coliseum. Games were to be Thursday and Saturday, which meant we left Hanover on Wednesday. Two more organic-chemistry labs to miss. I opened the books in my bag, but digested little over the next four days.

The Charlotte tournament hosts drove us around to show off their city. We were taken to a daytime mixer with Queens-University women. We called it a "look around."

The first game in the round of sixteen was with Manhattan College. As players we knew little about this New York City team. When we won, we were excited, and I was surprised. Were we really that good? One more game and we would be in the Final Four and have a chance to play against Wilt Chamberlain.

Our matchup for the right to play another weekend was Temple University, a Philadelphia powerhouse. They were led by Guy Rogers, who went on to a long career in the NBA. As the game progressed it was evident that this was the toughest team we had played all year. With Dartmouth down by ten points, I went into the game. First, a forward drove on me, stopped for a jump shot, and scored. Soon after he outjumped me for an offensive rebound and scored again. I was not to be the team's savior that night, nor was anyone else on the Dartmouth team. We lost to the team that went on to lose the National Championship game to the University of Kansas and Chamberlain the next weekend.

Our season had ended, but the Charlotte Dartmouth alumni were not finished with us. We were hosted at a series of parties into the early morning with barely time to meet a plane back to New York. The plane was a small DC-3 whose tail dropped to ground level as it landed. You had to walk uphill to exit the plane near the cockpit. We flew low in a strong wind. The bouncing and dipping made most of us nauseous. On landing I rushed up the sloping aisle, out the door to fresh air, and down the stairway to immediately leave "my cookies" from the night before on the runway.

Those years at Dartmouth balancing athletics and academics were challenging. I had made new friends, had tested my athletic and academic skills, had had some success in athletics, and had been admitted to medical school for my senior year. The challenge of balancing division-one athletics and premed studies required discipline, time management, and perseverance. I can't say those college years were the best of my life, but they helped me develop an understanding of what it takes to be successful in the pursuit of life goals.

All my freshmen teammates went on to successful adult lives: Tom Alley in business, Ed Hobbie in law, Nick Porcino and Micky Cohen in medicine. Rudy Laruso went on to play in the NBA for eleven years, ten of those years with the Minneapolis and Los Angeles Lakers, and was named to six all-star teams. Dave Gavitt, a reserve guard and my roommate, went on to be a highly successful college basketball coach, coach of the 1980 Olympic team, and founding commissioner of the Big East Athletic Conference. He has been inducted into the United States Basketball Hall of Fame in Hartford, Connecticut.

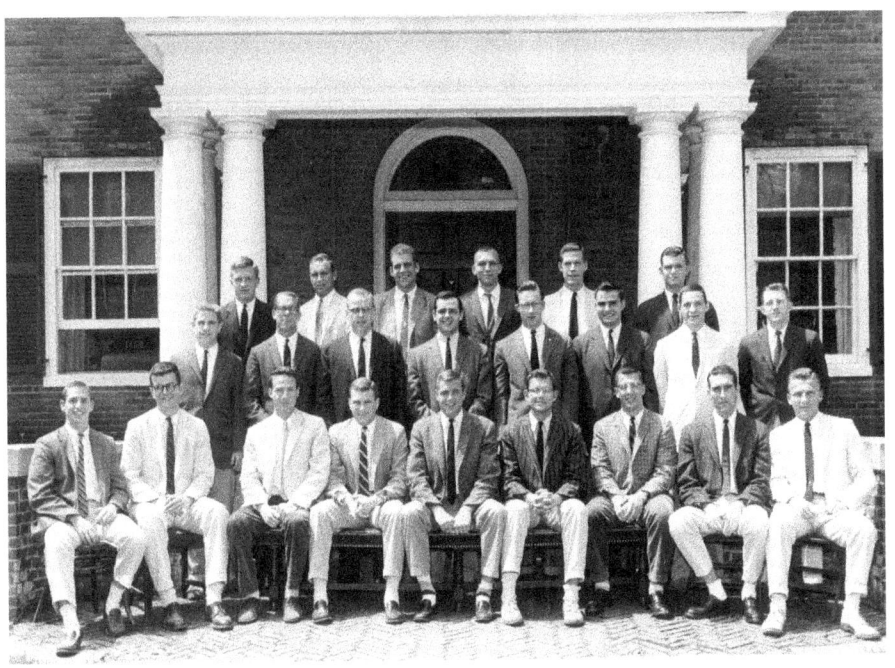

Casque and Gauntlet senior society, 1959. I am third from right in the back row. Ed Hobbie is second from the left in the front row.

CHAPTER NINE

Summer of 1961

As my six years in New Hampshire were drawing to a close, I felt my liberal-arts education needed some finishing touches. I had done most of what I set out to do in getting a good education; I had begun my trajectory in the medical field by finishing the first two years of medical school. I had tried out scientific research as a career for a year. But I hadn't broadened my understanding of the world outside of North America except for taking French language as a freshman. When Ida, my father's sister, declared she was going to make her first trip back to Sweden after emigrating with my Hanson grandparents as a child, I was intrigued. She would be the first person in the family to return after leaving in 1900.

I had not been out of the United States except to Canada. I had heard talk about Sweden all my life. Now there was the possibility of going to Europe and visiting relatives in Sweden with Ida. The 1960s were days of the Cold War with the Soviet Union. Europe was divided into East and West. Tension was building in Berlin over Germany's division and the economic disparities between the capitalist West and the communist East. I wanted to see for myself the Europe I had heard and read about.

As my research fellowship was drawing to a close in the spring of 1961, Robert Gosselin, my department head, announced he was going to present a paper at the August International Pharmacology meeting in Stockholm. Now I had two reasons to head for Sweden. I put the finishing touches on a research article, wrote up protocols for the cardiac-muscle-micropuncture technique I was working on, and prepared to make my way to Stockholm. It was early June and I had three weeks of vacation coming, which I could extend over the summer months, before I continued the third and fourth years of medical school at the University of Minnesota in September.

There was one problem — money. Medical students, and especially research fellows on their first grant, are not flush with ready cash, however student-loan payments could be delayed until after medical school graduation. The hot travel book of the time was *Europe on Five Dollars a Day*. I thought if I spent $10 a day including transportation, that $900 should last three months and still give me a thousand toward my last two years of medical school in Minnesota. At $300 a month from a NIH grant plus a night lab-tech position at the Mary Hitchcock Hospital, I was able to save the desired funds.

Many friends expressed interest in joining me, but in the end I headed off alone, hitchhiking to Montreal on June 9 for a flight to Shannon, Ireland on the tenth. The plane served Irish whiskey with the meals, and I joined other young travelers for the night flight. The North Atlantic chill in Shannon caught me by surprise, so I stopped at a secondhand store to buy a corduroy sport coat that kept me warm for the rest of the summer.

I hitchhiked to Killarney, walked the Gap of Dunloe, refused to kiss the Blarney Stone, was impressed with the ruins at Cashel, and took in more than one pint of beer in Dublin. I then flew to Scotland, hitched rides around Loch Lomond, stayed at youth hostels, visited Edinburgh, climbed Scafell Pike in England, walked the lake country of English poets, visited a classmate in Oxford, and stood for a performance of

Hamlet at the Stratford-on-Avon National Trust Theatre — all of which challenged my $10-a-day limit.

I could easily have spent weeks in London, but I was developing the rhythm of student travel and had a thirst to keep moving. Leaving behind new friends in London, I went to Amsterdam. On my first night, I went into a small cafe, looked at the menu in Dutch, and tried to communicate with the waiter, who was also the cook. Finally, I pointed to what looked like a hamburger. The next thing I knew, I was served raw ground meat on an open-faced bun. I was not familiar with "steak tartare" and tried to get the cook to fry it. He was indignant and obviously insulted. I choked down the raw meat, paid the bill, and made my way to the hostel.

One of my goals was to visit my boyhood friend, Bill Boeder, in Babenhausen, West Germany. He was a graduate metallurgical engineer who was a U.S. Army officer engaged in top-secret intelligence work close to the East German border. Bill and his wife, Barbara, introduced me to German beer, Rhine-Valley wines, and wiener schnitzel. We would unite again in August for a car trip to Sweden.

Soon I was off hitchhiking again to Paris, Tours, Bordeaux, and San Sebastian and Pamplona in Spain. By now I had developed some self-preservation techniques; I always carried cheese, salami, and bread and found night shelter when it was raining.

When the bulls began to run through the streets of Pamplona, I kept to the sidelines with the women and children. The cheap bullring seats were labeled "Sole." I knew that meant in the sun, but I was not prepared for the blistering afternoon heat. My fellow spectators produced just as much sweat as the bullfighters. I lost track of how many bulls were killed that afternoon. I followed the bulls as they were dragged into the streets, and I joined the crowds drinking wine from skins, singing songs, and eating food sold by street vendors.

Hitchhiking in Spain was intimidating at the time. Franco was the country's dictator after Spain's 1930s Civil War. His army was present in the towns, and police, usually in pairs, were stationed every few kilometers along the highways. Cars sped by my outstretched thumb, but an occasional truck stopped to offer me a bumpy, noisy, slow ride. It took an eternity to get past Zaragoza and eventually to Madrid.

My interest in Madrid was to experience a dictator's capital. There were many uniformed police, but the city bustled like any other large city. Dinner hour started at 11:00 p.m., flamenco dancing at midnight, and street activity continued into the early morning. The Prado Museum and its El Greco paintings impressed me as a young student who had spent most of his academic time studying the sciences.

From Barcelona, I went up the French valley to Grenoble and Chamonix where I was drawn to the mystique of Mont Blanc, the highest alp in Europe. Many dream of climbing mountains, and I was no exception. My previous White-Mountain experiences in New Hampshire were no match for the summer snowfields at the top of the cable car. Climbers with ropes, ice axes, and crampons were going out on narrow ridges that I passed by in the interest of self-preservation.

In Switzerland I was picked up by two girls driving a used Citroën 2 CV called a "Deux Chevaux," a French phrase for "two horsepower." The Citroën was an underpowered, light, thin metal-skinned, two-person car with plenty of air leaking through the doors, windows, and floorboards. My new companions didn't have definite plans, and we decided to head to Italy the next morning. Simplon was the closest mountain pass, and as we headed up I was sitting with my backpack and my knees near my chin in the cramped backseat space basically meant for luggage. The pass now has a tunnel that makes it safer, but less exciting.

As the climb became steeper, several cars alongside the road were steaming with overheated radiators. The little Citroën chugged along for a while, but the engine temperature was climbing. Downshifting gears didn't help much. Finally, it was obvious that we were overloaded, and I was the culprit. Reluctantly, I volunteered to get out. Traveling with two college-age women was not unpleasant, and they were looking for someone to give them direction. I was disappointed, but with the lightened load, they took off up the pass, and I did not see them again the rest of the summer. Now I was back to hitchhiking on a mountain-pass road where cars were failing and no one wanted to risk the weight of an extra body on the way up the mountainside.

Finally, a motorcycle stopped. The German driver had a cycle right out of a war movie — maybe the First World War — with spoked wheels, a smoky exhaust, and a putt-putt-sounding engine. The prospects didn't look good, but the driver was willing. There wasn't a real seat on the back fender, and he had to dig into a side bag for some stirrups that somehow attached near the rear axle for my feet. This machine looked like it would have had trouble getting one person over the pass, and now we were two. I settled into my position, leaning forward with my backpack, with both feet on the ground to balance the bike, while my benefactor kicked the starter. After several attempts, it started. He gunned the engine, and then ran alongside. As the bike picked up speed, he hopped on, and we were off. Slowly, we struggled up the mountain, but kept moving, like the little engine that could. As we reached the top, I felt relieved as we planed over the pass only to realize that we had to go down the other side.

Now it became evident that my driver was a true biker. The little engine that could was now a power house and the winding descent a Formula-One racetrack. He was in his element. We leaned into curves, cut across lanes, and seemed to pick up speed with each bend in the road. I had the feeling approaching cars were slowing down just to watch the accident that was about to happen. Minutes went by. I thought the bends in the road would never end. My stomach churned.

I did my best to hang on, balance my pack, keep my feet on the stirrups, control my bladder, and breathe. When we reached a small village and the road leveled out, he slowed down, stopped, grinned, and indicated that was as far as he was going. I expressed my thanks and sat down by the roadside shaken, but glad to be alive. I resolved to never ride on a motorcycle again, but that resolve didn't last long.

During my first experience in Italy, I took in the highlights — the northern lakes, Pisa, Florence, Assisi, Rome, and Venice. I was impressed with the Roman Forum and Coliseum, the fountains, St. Peter's Square, and the speed of cars on the freeways.

The more I traveled, the more intriguing getting past the Iron Curtain became. Vienna was known to be an entry point into Hungary, a Soviet satellite at the time. At the Hungarian embassy I was told a tourist visit was possible if I left my passport for ten days and paid all expenses in advance. I didn't want to wait, and tie up most of my remaining money with a month still to go. I decided instead to head back to Germany for a car trip to Sweden with my friend, Bill Boeder, and his brother.

Riding in a car with friends was less challenging than begging for rides, meeting new people several times a day, and waiting for hours along dusty roadsides. We headed north through the Netherlands along the Zuiderzee into Denmark, visiting Kronborg Castle (Shakespeare's setting for *Hamlet*), and ferrying to Almhult in southern Sweden where the Boeder brothers had family to meet. The family fed me a big dinner and put me on a train to Stockholm. When I arrived, the hostels were closed for the night, so I slept under a railroad bridge out of the rain. I was dry, but trains passed overhead most of the night shaking the ground under me with deafening noise.

I was planing to meet my aunt Ida. The next morning I found out she was in Sollefteå, about 500 miles north, near her childhood home. She had a busy schedule planned for the next week, including family gatherings that I was expected to attend. I also wanted to visit my mother's side of the family in Essunga, which was in the opposite direction in western Sweden near Göteborg. And there was the pharmacology conference in Stockholm, which was one of the two original reasons for my whole trip.

These activities were going to take ten days or more, so the next thing I did was to head to the Polish Embassy, the diplomatic link between Sweden and the Soviet Union. I could make a tourist trip to Leningrad (now called St. Petersburg), Moscow, Warsaw, and Berlin, but I needed to leave my passport for ten days to get a visa and to pay for all travel and accommodations in advance. I knew the drill and was ready to sign up. Counting my residual traveler's checks — this was long before credit and debit cards — I figured the only way I could make it was to rent a Russian car and camp. Campsites were less than two rubles a day (exchange was artificially pegged at one ruble to the dollar), and a car rental less than $100 for a week. I would enter through Finland and go by train to Leningrad, drive to Moscow, and take the train from Moscow through Poland to Berlin. It all sounded good, even though I would be traveling alone and using up most of my funds. I put my money down, left my passport, and headed north to meet Ida and the Swedish relatives.

The next days were filled with new faces, coffee, and food. I had a hard time remembering all the names, who was related to whom, and how they were related to the American Hansons. All was going well until they found out I did not have my passport. The relatives were sure that I wouldn't get it back from the Polish Embassy and I would be stuck in Sweden indefinitely in their charge. And then on August 13 the connection between East and West Berlin was closed. Two days later the East Germans began building a wall that was to last the next twenty-eight years. Berlin was an international city isolated in the heart of East Germany, the result of political accommodations after Germany lost World War ll.

Ida and my Swedish relatives were distraught. I certainly could not go to the Soviet Union under these circumstances. They wanted me to go immediately to Stockholm to get my passport back. Forget the money. I can't say I wasn't concerned, but my travel plans seemed more intriguing each day. I had been on the road for over two months, and the relatives' reactions seemed to make the challenge more inviting. I went on to visit the Larson relatives in western Sweden and came back to Stockholm to meet my department chief for three days of pharmacology meetings. I attended the professor's talk, stayed a second day, and then split for the Polish Embassy.

The night before I was to leave for Finland, I met a man from California, Sig Jacobs, who had grown up as a Jew in Warsaw during the 1930s. He spoke Polish and knew some Russian. He was insistent on joining me for the ten-day trip. The idea of a traveling partner was desirable, but who was he? How did he find me? Was he an agent of some government or just an interested traveler like me? He was more than twice my age, much more experienced, and had language capabilities that would be useful. I didn't think he had a chance of getting a visa the same day we would be leaving, but I agreed to meet him at the embassy in the morning, where I was expecting to pick up my passport and travel vouchers. When the Polish agent heard our request, he looked puzzled and definitely not encouraging. He agreed to take our request to some higher authority, took my new partner's passport, and disappeared. Nothing happened for over an hour. Finally he returned and said we were both approved to leave that night. I was surprised! This older man, whom I had met just twelve hours earlier was granted a visa in an hour and was to be my companion on an uncertain trip, to places of international news coverage. Was he an undercover agent? I wasn't sure then. I am still not sure.

CHAPTER TEN

Behind the Iron Curtain

The night ferry from Sweden to Finland landed in Abo (pronounced obo), yet when Sig and I boarded the train to Helsinki we were leaving from Turku. The same city has both Swedish and Finnish names depending on which country made the map. As we got closer to the border with Russia, we got more inside information on what to expect. "In Moscow they will buy the clothes off your back," other travelers told us. "Bring several pairs of Levi jeans." I brought what I had in my pack and on my back, and we headed for the Russian wide-track train at the Helsinki station. Russian rail tracks were and still are wider than the European-standard gauge, a residual fear of overland invasion from the West.

There was little joviality on the train. Was this business as usual, or did the passengers' moods reflect the tension and uncertainty about the events unfolding in Berlin? In Leningrad (now called St. Petersburg) the Russian tourist bureau, Intourist, seemed to be expecting us, but they wanted more money. The Volga car I had rented needed to be returned from Moscow to Leningrad. Since we were not making a round trip, Intourist demanded several hundred dollars more. When I explained we didn't have the cash, they said we could spend our ten days in Leningrad and then return to Helsinki. Without a car, camping was out of the question. We argued for a hotel room for our prepaid camping fee. Somehow they bought our plight and put us up in a business hotel in the city center. Shortly after we arrived, two young men who said they were students practicing English, introduced themselves and offered to show us around. Now I was surrounded by three people who possibly were not telling me exactly who they were or why they wanted to follow me.

Leningrad was still recovering from the war. I was not impressed with the city known as the Venice of Russia. The canals were empty and the roads and boulevards in poor repair. We saw lots of street sweepers and stalls selling cigarettes and piroshkis (Russian meat pies), but not much else. The Hermitage hadn't been opened since World War ll and was under repair. There were workmen around a concert hall where we were prohibited from witnessing a rehearsal and were told there were no performances scheduled.

A few blocks from our hotel was St. Isaac's Cathedral, the centerpiece of Imperial Russian Orthodox churches in old St. Petersburg. It had been turned into a museum that was exhibiting recent communist accomplishments. Our "English-learning students" offered to take us to one of their homes. When we arrived after a bus ride, they checked with the family who said they were not interested in entertaining any foreign visitors. Our volunteer student guides found several ways of keeping us from doing what we thought would be interesting.

We still wanted to get to Moscow, Poland, and Berlin. We learned there was a daily evening flight from Leningrad to Moscow, however Intourist representatives did not want us to leave the city. On a Sunday morning, my industrious partner tried to convince the clerk on call that we had been approved the day before to take that evening's flight to Moscow. No record of such approval was found after an extensive search. We told our sad story about the car, our inability to camp, our dwindling funds, and our prepaid train ticket from Moscow to Berlin. Finally, the bewildered duty clerk issued us two tickets for the flight we wanted. We had to give him the flight and seat numbers we knew were available. These negotiations sounded unusual and maybe fishy. My partner spoke some Russian and much of our dealing was conducted outside of my full understanding. My partner had skills or connections that I would not have had traveling alone.

The hour flight to Moscow was smooth and uneventful. We got off the plane about 10:00 p.m., where an Intourist agent was checking off each passenger. When we came up, he couldn't find our names. Their system had broken down. He was agitated and called for help. Now we had several agents on our case. They asked where we were staying, and we told them we were planning to stay in a hotel for Eastern European businessmen that we knew charged less than two rubles a night. But when they checked, there were no reservations in our names. They wanted to put us in a tourist hotel at twenty-five rubles a night. We said we just didn't have the money. Eventually someone called a taxi, and we were driven to the cheap hotel. For about $1.60 a night and about $.30 for breakfast, the hotel became our home for the next several days.

The hotel was near a subway station, and we began exploring the center of the evil empire the following morning. Lenin and Stalin were laid out in their tombs on Red Square. The Kremlin was bristling with guards who made sure we didn't step on the grass. The GUM department store facing Red Square was touted as the prime jewel of Soviet merchandising, and yet displayed nothing of value to us — only shoddy goods, few shoppers, and surly salespeople. It seemed the "Great Red Menace" was a third-world country as far as manufactured consumer goods were concerned.

The iconic St. Basil's Cathedral at one end of Red Square was closed, fenced off, and in severe disrepair. A Soviet exhibition outside the city featuring ethnic and cultural regions seemed to be a promotional display of what was to come rather than what had been accomplished. They did have something to brag about in displays related to space and the Sputnik satellite. When I returned thirty years later in 1991, the Russian flag flew over the Kremlin, the bodies were gone, and St. Basil's Cathedral was open and repaired.

Many young Russians were interested in our clothes. We had no Levi jeans, but we were still approached about selling almost anything we were wearing: trousers, shirts, hats, jackets — any outside clothing made in the West was desirable. I sold most everything I owned, replacing the essentials with whatever I could trade or find in shops. The corduroy sportcoat I bought the first day in Ireland now had a Muscovite owner.

One day a Russian about my age insisted on having my beat-up cardigan sweater. It was well worn, ragged, and necessary for cool nights. I tried to dissuade him but he was insistent. He offered me a price I couldn't refuse, and he was off with his purchase. The next morning, when I came up out of the subway near Red Square, he was waiting for me. He tried to tell me that I had cheated him, the sweater was worthless. I gladly returned his rubles, and I had my worn but warm sweater back.

Sig and I looked forward to a train ride through the Russian countryside after visiting two major cities. The farm fields were large and mostly devoid of people or any evidence of farm equipment. Occasionally, we passed a commune with farm sheds and a few pieces of machinery. There didn't seem to be much activity, and the fields were often barren.

The train passed through Minsk, the capital of what was then called White Russia (Russia Alba). The region reclaimed its earlier name, Belarus, after the Soviet Union dissolved. We had planned a two-night stay and started to explore. An Intourist guide wanted to show us around and tout their progress. The main thoroughfare was lined with dull two-to-six-story, grey stucco, Soviet-style buildings on both sides for more than a mile. One block back on either side was brick-and-stone rubble. Minsk was a city of 500,000 people before World War ll. It had been mostly abandoned and destroyed by German attacks. Sixteen years after the war's end, I doubt that more than 10,000 people called Minsk home. The contrast between the rebuilt main street and the rest of the city was stark and unsettling. For the first time I experienced the complete devastation that can come with war.

Leaving Minsk, we came to Brest where the Russian-gauge track changes to European gauge before entering Poland. We were spirited away to a station house so we could not observe the process. After a few hours, we reboarded and headed for Warsaw. As soon as we crossed the border, the farms were green with small fields of variable crops, and we saw many people and horses working the fields. The contrast between Russia and Poland shouldn't have been surprising. The large communes of the Soviet Union definitely had not taken hold in its satellite country.

Warsaw also provided a marked contrast to the Soviet cities. Except for one government tower in an area that was probably the Jewish neighborhood that became the notorious Warsaw ghetto, the city was alive with activity (no one would tell me exactly where the ghetto had been located). We witnessed an active nightlife, enjoyed the food and drink, and remarked on the vibrant commercial activity compared to Moscow and Leningrad.

The final leg of this journey behind the Iron Curtain was an uneventful train ride from Warsaw through Poland and the East German countryside into Berlin. It had been three weeks since the East Germans closed the border and started building a wall separating East and West Berlin. Potential escapees had been apprehended, and several had been shot and killed.

We rolled into the East Berlin station in the evening. It was dark, and few people remained on the train. As we got off, a uniformed East Berlin police officer, was checking passports. When he saw we were Americans, he pointed to a set of stairs and gurgled some words that indicated we needed to move. Up the stairs was an empty elevated train. Another officer motioned for us to get on. The train with several cars was completely empty. The doors shut, and the train took off. Usually we could get some advance information from other travelers about what to expect, but in this case we were flying blind. Somewhere, out in the dark a wall was being built, and we guessed we were going over it. All of a sudden there were street lights and people out walking. We stopped near Kurfurstendamm, the main commercial street in West Berlin. Somewhat shaken, we asked directions to the refugee hostel. It had been a main refuge earlier that summer for East Germans fleeing west. Now it was nearly deserted, and we had the place mostly to ourselves.

Sig and I had been together for nearly two weeks. Our tolerance for each other was getting thin. He was interested in the infamous nightlife in West Berlin at the time while I was more interested in experiencing and understanding what was really going on in the divided city. We amicably parted company, and I was on my own again.

My solitude did not last long. I met a Tunisian with a Vespa motor scooter. We were able to communicate in French, and shortly we were off to Checkpoint Charlie on Friedrichstrasse. Crossing from East to West Berlin for tourists was possible only through this point. Staggered barricades had been set up to prevent anyone trying to make a run for it. Hundreds of uniformed police and soldiers on each side were peering at one another through binoculars. Almost no one was moving from one side to the other. With his Tunisian passport and mine from the United States, we got though after several checks of our papers by American officers and then, on the other side, by East German police. Once through the zigzag barricades, we were free to roam.

At that time Western governments were manipulating the German mark exchange rate. For the equivalent of five dollars, we could get forty dollars worth of East German marks. We were off to the races, buying clothes I needed, a camera for my father, and whatever looked like a bargain to my Tunisian friend. The goods went under my riding seat on the Vespa scooter, which was a real seat as opposed to the Simplon-Pass motorcycle. Food was good by our standards and cheap. We ate well, had good wine, and made some friends. We frequented a wine stube a block from Checkpoint Charlie near a police barracks and right next to a Russian artillery battery poised for action. We were careful not to provoke anyone looking official.

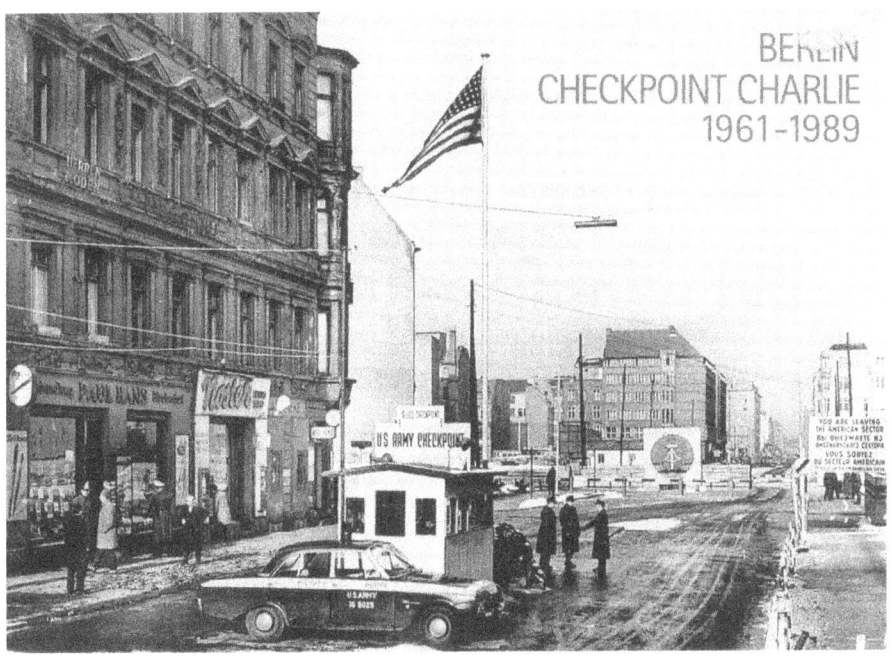

Checkpoint Charlie as it appeared in 1961
In the distance were the Russian artillery and East German wine stuben.
(Unable to identify source of graphic.)

After several days of sleeping in the West Berlin hostel and spending days and evenings in East Berlin, we decided it was time to head west to Hanover by the only route available. At the time Berlin was a four-powers international city deep in East Germany. The autobahn access had been interrupted in the late 1940s after the war, leading to a Berlin airlift by the Western governments. But now a single autobahn was open from Berlin in the east to Hanover in the west. With our under-seat space filled with his purchases and my filled pack on my back, we started off.

Riding on the Vespa on open roads was different from riding on Berlin's city streets. The road was flat, had no sharp curves, and our speed could not have been more than 40 mph. Every crossroad had two or three police guards, and police cars continued to pass us off and on. All was going well for about forty minutes until the scooter began to sputter, jerk a few times, and die. We had run out of gas.

No car was about to stop for us on this heavily policed road. Luckily, no police car passed. Finally, a motorcycle stopped. We gestured our plight, and he offered to take one of us to get gas. I was not excited to be designated, but my Tunisian friend said he didn't want to leave his scooter.

Off we went, retracing our autobahn path to a crossroad leading to a small village. The cyclist explained my situation to the police, while I kept my mouth shut. We were waved through and found an auto-repairman who poured some gas into two liter-sized milk bottles. Now it was time to pay, and I blurted out, "How much?" in English. The attendant was shocked, became excited, and motioned for us to leave. I had exchanged all my German marks, so I offered U.S. dollars. He was so anxious to get us moving he would take nothing, not even the marks offered by our good Samaritan motorcyclist. Back on the cycle, we went past the police at the crossroad, and up to the Vespa, where we filled the tank and were off to Hanover again.

BEHIND THE IRON CURTAIN

I don't remember much about Hanover, about hitchhiking to Amsterdam, or flying to Montreal. I do remember crossing the U.S. border in Vermont, entering a small restaurant, and ordering a hamburger, fries, and a Coke. Back in my home country, I ate our signature meal. It was a big disappointment, even worse than the steak tartare in Amsterdam.

Looking back, the summer of 1961 exposed me to European cultures, to my Scandinavian heritage, and to the major international conflicts of the twentieth century on a personal basis. It gave me confidence that I could make decisions and take risks without consulting others. I could travel with strangers and experience new things with a minimum of fear. I could do unusual things others might reject and learn from them. It changed my views on politics and conflict between nations. I came back more tolerant of diverse opinions and behaviors, more liberal in politics, and less tolerant of armed conflict between individuals and nations.

Family and Work

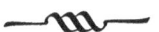

CHAPTER ELEVEN

Finding Love

Why were our sixth-grade teachers teaching us to dance? The boys wanted to shoot basketballs at the gym's low rims. The girls already knew the steps. There were two girls in the class who were as athletic as any boy. They played softball with us during recess and at lunch time. Neither was the last to be chosen when sides were picked.

One day, when the bell rang for school to start, a girl, it could have been Nancy DuFour, asked if she could take my picture with Diane Bouchard, one of the softball players. When she asked us to hold hands, I knew something was up — Diane became my first girlfriend. When the picture was passed around, we were the same height. Diane looked mature and confident, and I looked bewildered. This was a new experience, and I was at a loss. Parents scheduled boy-girl parties that spring, and I became part of someone else's plan. Summer came just in time to save me.

The next fall Diane and I started junior high in a new school several miles away. Schoolbuses were not available, so our parents organized car pools. For the next six years, Diane and I rode to school together. However our budding romance dissolved with the influx of new boy talent.

At five-foot-four inches, I wasn't a runt, but a six-foot-two classmate, who shaved each morning and played center on all basketball teams was the athletic hero of the class. Hormones raged, acne popped out, and erections came at inopportune times. Diane found another boyfriend and I grew three inches a year for the next three years. My view of the school world and of myself changed considerably.

Friday-night parties were another adult plan for getting boys and girls together. About once a month, Ramsey Junior High School was opened for dancing to recorded music in the girls' gym, for food in the cafeteria, and for basketball in the boys' gym. The boys hung out in the obvious place. But by ninth grade, some of us spent some time dancing the Lindy Hop. (I use the same steps for any fast dance sixty-five years later.) Slow music gave some couples a chance to get closer and more intimate as the lights dimmed.

One day, when we were in ninth grade, a bright, beautiful girl in Mrs. Allen's English class asked if I would go to a fall picnic with her and some friends. I was assured parents would transport us back and forth, and she would provide the food. Who could say no to this attractive classmate? Her name was Gail Taylor.

The picnic was near Minnehaha Creek Falls (of Longfellow fame) in what was called the deer pen — a wooded valley where the Minneapolis Park Board had confined stray deer. The valley had been scoured out by a creek for thousands of years. It was a place where grade-schoolers went to search for strange-looking prehistoric sea fossils. It also was a secluded place for a group picnic. I was learning the dating game and was impressed with Gail and her friends.

Some months later, one of Gail's friends, Faye Kirkness, asked if I would go to a house party with her. Once at the party, we danced, ate, and I was having a good time when she informed me that I would not be going home with her. She was going home with her former boyfriend, and I was going home with his date, Gail Taylor. I was smitten with Gail, but too shy to ask her on a date. I was just fourteen and a birthday away from having a driver's license. Gail lived two miles away, and a bicycle date was not cool. By the time I had more confidence, she was busy with older, more sophisticated boys who could drive. That was the last time I took Gail home for the next ten years.

As spring approached that ninth-grade year, I was invited to a school dance, another girl-ask-boy event. One of the girls in our church youth choir, Jane Ellingson, asked if I would go with her. This wasn't an authorized church dance, but I expect our mothers compared notes. She was a year younger, and a Luther-League regular. She and I dated regularly throughout high school and off and on during college for the next seven years. We attended colleges in different parts of the country and gradually moved apart. When I came back to Minnesota, she was teaching school in California.

The medical school at Dartmouth was part of a complex then called the Mary Hitchcock Hospital and Clinics. The associated nursing school drew student nurses, most of whom were interested in finding a medical-student partner. If you weren't already paired with someone, there were plenty of matchmakers in the all-male medical school and all-female nursing school. By this time I was six foot four. Alice Vadarkis was five foot one. We were an unusual couple on the dance floor. She skied well, and we were hard to beat on the tennis courts with my long arms at the net and her strong ground strokes. But when I completed my six years in Hanover, I headed for a summer in Europe, and Alice pursued a nursing job and life in Seattle where her brother lived.

New Hampshire and Vermont were sparsely populated in the early twentieth century. Dartmouth Medical School offered the first two years of instruction in basic medical sciences and then students transferred to large city medical centers for the remaining two clinical years.

After considering my options, I decided it was time to get back to my Minnesota roots. The University of Minnesota had accepted me as a transfer student for the fall of 1961. When friends ask what drew me back to Minnesota, I said I needed to finish medical school somewhere, and it was time to think about finding a wife. Barbara Krampitz, the wife of the Lutheran minister at Dartmouth, when asked why she married her husband, David, said, "You marry the person you are dating when you both are ready to get married."

Back in Minnesota, I found a rooming house, started a surgical rotation, and resumed hunting and fishing. I also made a call to Gail, my ninth-grade picnic date. Through the years I had double-dated with Gail who went out with an older friend, Bill Boeder, who had use of a car. She was someone I wanted to contact when I returned to Minnesota. Then, there was the big question — was she available? She had dated more than one of my friends, so I knew some of her comings and goings. I knew that she had attended the University of Minnesota and left Minneapolis to teach school in California.

When I called her in the fall of 1961, one of her four brothers answered their rotary-dial phone that sat on a small shelf behind their center hall stairway. (I later found out her father never answered because it was never for him.) "Gail's not home. She is teaching school in California." I would have to wait another year.

California schools recessed for the summer in the spring of 1962. I had heard from friends that Gail was back in town, so I made another call. A brother answered and called for her. When she didn't answer, he said, "She must have already gone to the wedding." I was too shocked to ask, "Whose wedding?"

Weeks went by. Finally a good friend assured me it was not Gail's wedding, so I called again. A brother answered. "She's in the living room. I'll get her." When Gail came to the phone, we had a nice, slowly developing five-minute conversation. When I asked if she was available to go out, she said, "Not really." Then she went on to tell me I had called just as she and her fiancé were in the living room telling her parents about their marriage plans. At that point she was called back to the living room, our call ended, and I exhaled.

Many weeks later, I received a note with a phone number at my rooming house. I recognized the number as Gail's. We had another slowly developing conversation about her trip back to Minnesota, about her new suburban teaching job, and about the fact she was no longer engaged. I was planning a trip west to look at internships. When we met for lunch, she gave me a record album to give to her former roommate, Rachel Olson, in San Francisco. That seemed like a harmless request, and I agreed.

When I contacted Rachel between internship interviews, she invited me for dinner. I gave her the Drinking Gourd record, and after dinner we went off to see the town. She was from Mankato, Minnesota, had similar midwest experiences, and our conversations went on into the night. The next day we went to the zoo. I can't remember what we did in the next few days, but when I left town, I was several days off schedule, lighter in my wallet, and had a new interest. I took the bus to Portland and Seattle where I had interviews and returned with just enough money to get back to Minneapolis. I had $.34 in my pocket when I arrived at my rooming house at 6:00 a.m. to start a new medical rotation at 8:00.

Back in Minnesota while I was writing to Rachel, Gail and I had several dates. One night we were going to a party with her new work colleagues. As we entered my old 1952 Dodge sedan with power-glide transmission, she remembered we were supposed to bring our own beverage. I went back into her parents' house to get a bourbon bottle she had put in her father's liquor cabinet over the refrigerator. I went into the kitchen and, as I was reaching for the bottle, her father, Glen, came around the corner and said, "First you take my daughter out, then you come back to take my liquor." Our encounter at the liquor cabinet became a story he loved to tell for years to come.

That night was a turning point in our relationship. We danced, we talked, and when it came time to part at her doorstep, we kissed for the first time. Was it the warm fall evening, or the familiarity I was developing in the Taylor house, or was it the spirits in the bottle that brought us together?

I was invited to Gail's home for a family Thanksgiving dinner. On a walk to Lake Harriet afterward, Gail said Rachel was coming for Christmas and was planning to see me. She asked if I was planning to see her? I had been interested in Gail since our ninth-grade picnic date. Now that she was interested in me, I was not going to lose my chances. The next day I wrote the necessary letter to Rachel.

By Christmastime Gail and I were phoning daily and seeing each other whenever we were free. (This was long before email and texting.) I was invited for dinner on Christmas Eve. The Taylor family was gathered around their large dining-room table. All the Swedish specialties were laid out — meatballs and gravy, rutabaga, mashed potatoes, lingonberries, and, of course, lutefisk. When Gail's mother, Hildur, saw that I ate my lutefisk with drawn butter and allspice, I think she felt I would be a good marriage prospect. By the time Gail came to New Jersey to meet my family for New Year's Eve, we knew where we were headed.

Some time in February, around Valentine's Day, we decided to get married. We called her parents, and Hildur answered. When we hinted what was up, she called out, "Glen, you better come to the phone." I told him, "I'm holding your daughter's hand. Can I have it?" Somewhat confused, he gave the phone back to Hildur.

The Taylor family planned our wedding for June at the nearby Swedish Lutheran Mount Olivet Church, which had the largest Lutheran congregation in the country at the time. June was also my graduation month from medical school and the last days were intense. My family decided to hold the groom's luncheon on graduation day, a Saturday. I attended the graduation ceremony that evening, and we were married the next afternoon. My dad, Rod Anderson, the best man, and I played golf in the morning and returned just in time for the wedding.

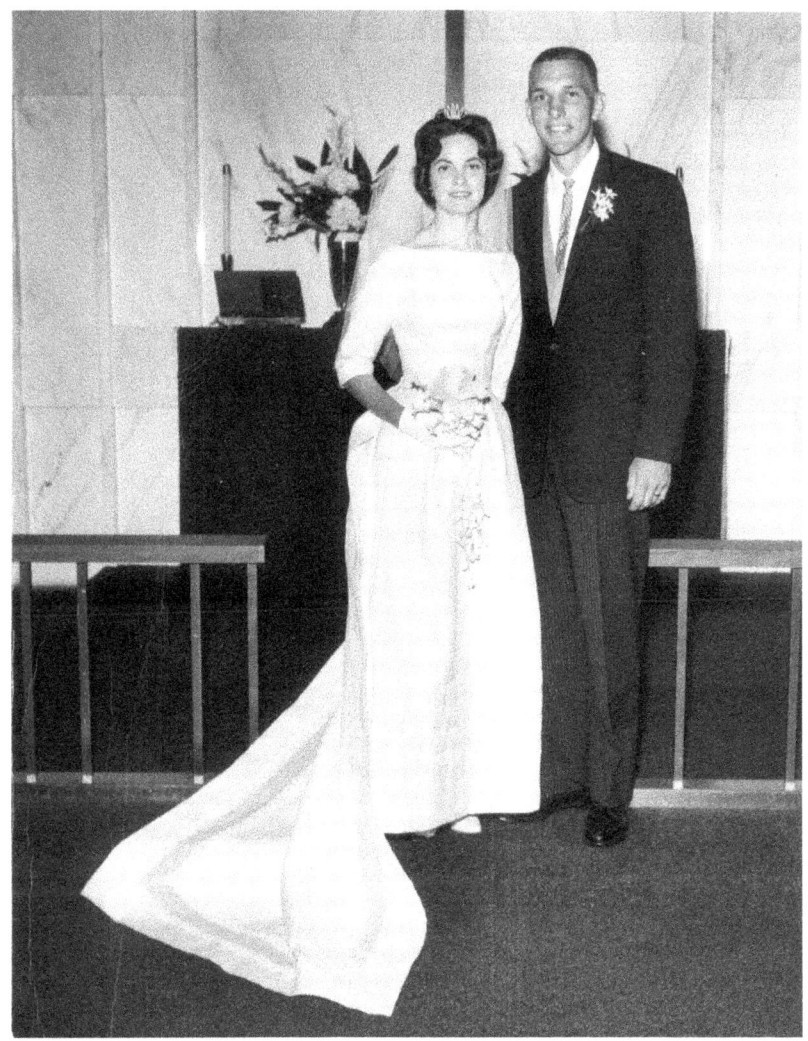

June 16, 1963

The reception was in the Taylors' backyard. Glen had prepared two cattle-watering tanks with ice for a hundred bottles of champagne. Gail's youngest brother, Greg (later called by his middle name Bert), and his young cousins made rounds of the tables making sure they all had enough champagne. Glen required them to only open bottles when a table requested one. They loved popping the corks, and the next morning there were dozens in the neighbor's rain gutters.

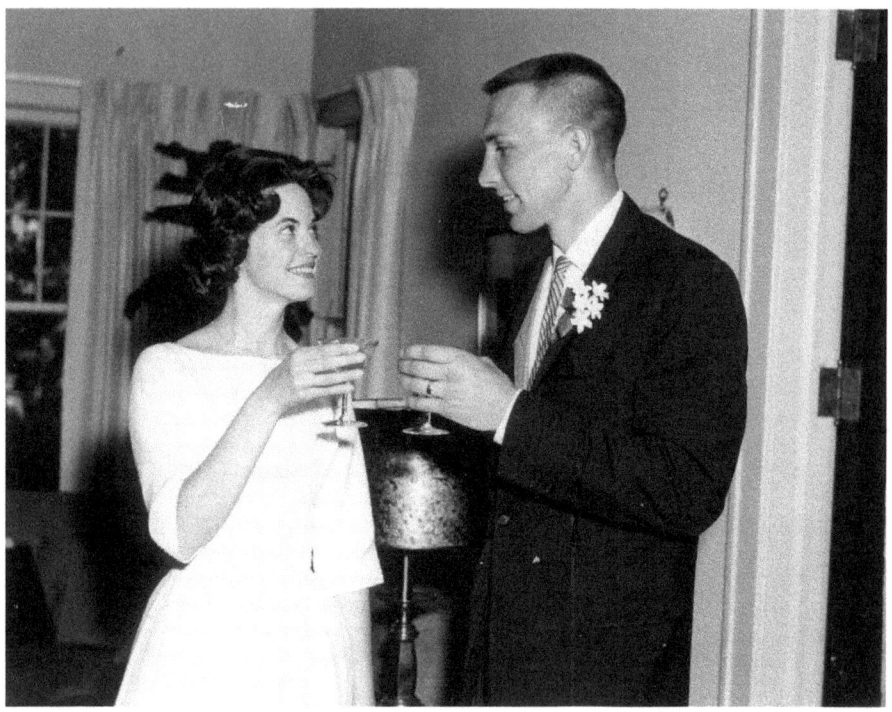

Champagne reception

We were expected to leave before the guests. Just before we were leaving, Gordie Sundin took me aside and said, "Stuie, you have married the smartest and most beautiful girl in our Washburn class." Later we learned that many of our friends stayed past midnight. They said it was the best party they had ever attended. One couple claimed that was the very last time they drank champagne or any other kind of alcohol.

FINDING LOVE

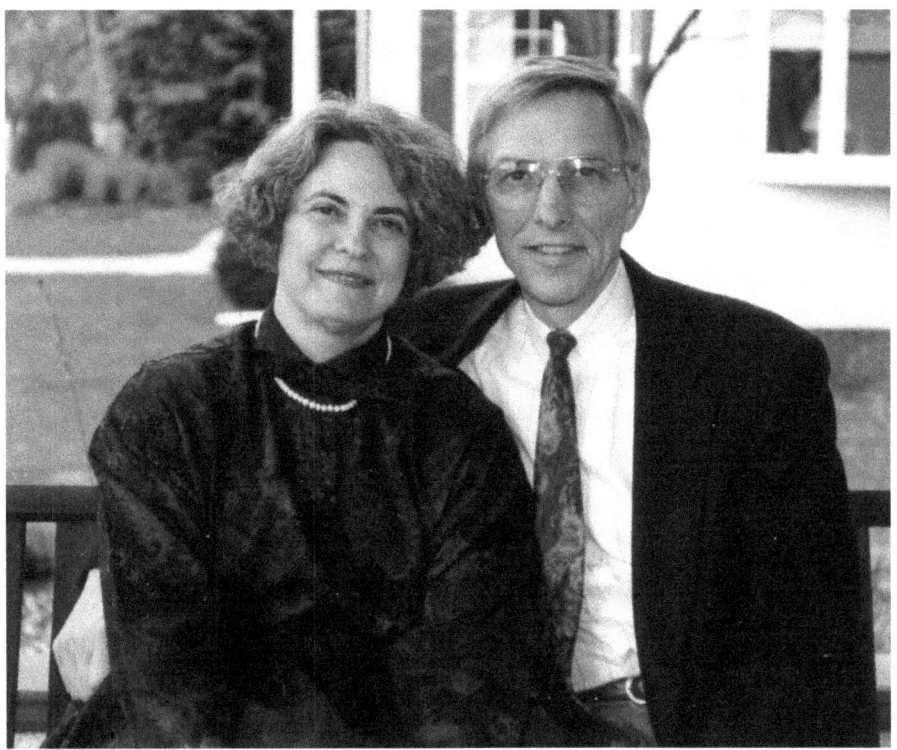

1992

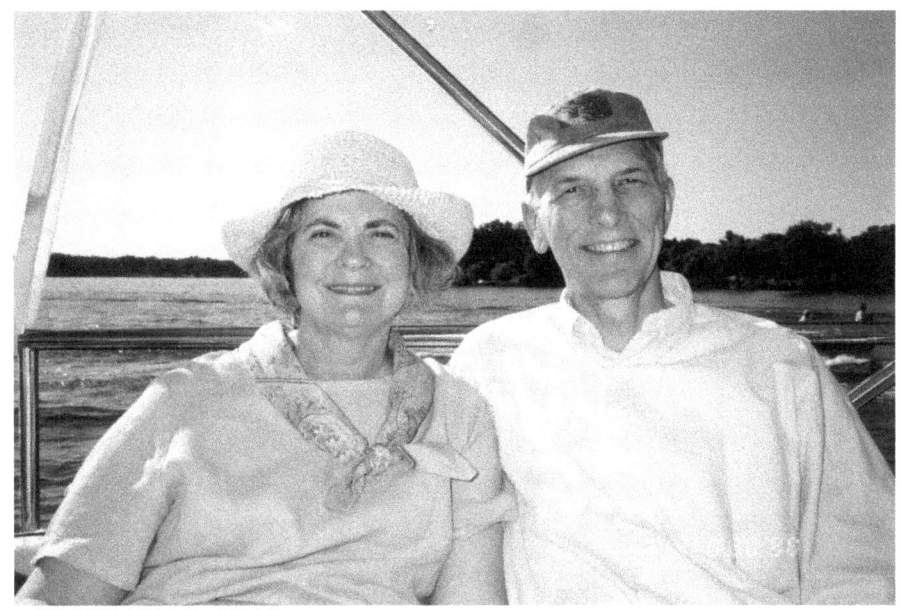

2002

CHAPTER TWELVE

The General

Minneapolis General Hospital was begun in the nineteenth century as a city hospital for the contagious and the poor. Quarantine for people with infectious diseases was common before antibiotics and successful immunizations. My father was admitted there as a young man with diphtheria in the 1920s. The hospital was also a place for the indigent who did not have access to the privately supported ethnic hospitals built by northern European immigrant Protestant and Catholic religious communities. In 1963 "The General," as it was called, had developed into a major U.S. teaching hospital for physicians and nurses. When I applied for a medical internship, the salary was $75 a month, but by the time I started, the salary had risen to $150 per month. As a newly married physician, I was starting at the bottom.

Orientation week started the last week in June where thirty-nine interns were primed for a year of medical submersion. We broke into thirteen three-member teams. Each team would rotate to a different medical service every four weeks. Doug Kjellsen, Jerry Lane, and I would be sharing call every third night for the next year. Sleeping rooms were arranged so no roommates were on call the same night. I rarely saw my roommate who was on another team, but his story will come later.

We received white pants and uniform shirts with our names embroidered over the left breast pocket. With stethoscopes around our necks and reflex hammers in our pockets, we were ready to ply our new trade. Our team's first assignment was the locked psychiatry ward located in one of the connected buildings, some of which had serviced the community for nearly a century. The chief ward nurse gave us an orientation, assigned us to patients, and turned us loose. An attending psychiatrist would supervise us several times a week and would be on call anytime we needed help. A resident physician would be available each day. It all sounded reasonable, and the first day we went to work getting to know our assigned patients.

I drew the first night call. After eating an evening meal of kitchen leftovers in the staff dining room, I took the elevator to the psychiatry floor of the annex building and let myself into the locked ward to meet the swing-shift nurse and to see how things were settling down for the evening. All was quiet. I went to my new sleeping room directly off the house staff lounge in another building, read a little, and turned off the light. This wasn't my first experience with medical night call, but it was the first time I would be the first in line.

At eleven o'clock just as the nursing shift was changing, we received a call to get ready for a "direct admission," which I later learned meant that the patient was bypassing the emergency room and coming directly to the psych floor. (We called the emergency receiving area the ER. Only later did it graduate to department status along with the development of emergency medicine as a medical specialty.)

I rousted myself out of bed, rushed to the annex, directed the elevator to the seventh floor, let myself into the unit, and waited with the nurse. In a few minutes we saw the elevator coming up. We gave permission for the door to open on the locked ward and out poured four muscular policemen and a struggling, expletive-yelling, dirty, unshaven male wrapped in a white straightjacket. It was like a scene from an old movie. (Although this happened before the release of Jack Nicholson's *One Flew Over the Cuckoo's Nest*.)

What were we going to do now? I looked at the nurse and before either of us could say anything, the police unwrapped our thrashing, yelling, spitting patient and left.

When I asked the nurse what we should do, she said, "I guess you need to take his history, do a physical exam, and get him to bed." Then she went back to her station and signed out for the night. To my surprise, the patient calmed down, told me his story, let me examine him, and went to bed without further problems.

The psych ward introduced Doug, Jerry, and me to the world of mental health. There were only a few medications that were effective at the time. Thorazine was just becoming available, talk therapy was so time consuming it could only be applied to select cases, and the warehousing of severe cases in state hospitals was common. The unit at Minneapolis General was a crisis center that frequently discharged patients back to the streets where they were picked up by police, thus continuing the cycle.

Another night Jerry Lane's patient, a depressed man in his early twenties, pushed out a heavily grated window screen and jumped. He landed in a basement-window well and somehow survived. No orthopedic or surgery ward would take him, so we managed his fractured pelvis, broken arm and leg, and severe bruises, and watched for internal bleeding on our psych ward.

Another morning I arrived to find a maintenance person mopping up blood in the men's bathroom. One of Doug Kjellsen's patients had tried to slit his throat the night before. His objective was the same, but he had been more successful than the jumper. Such was our introduction to our internship, to psychiatry, to "The General," and to our chosen profession.

My interest was in general medicine. General practice only required a year's internship until you were licensed and turned loose. Several of our intern colleagues went on to practice general medicine for over fifty years. I could see that general practice was declining and specialty practice growing. I then decided internal medicine was a logical track to follow, and I was excited when our medicine rotation came around.

General Hospital was H-shaped with the medical and surgical wards on the west side of the building. Medicine was on the second floor above the emergency room, and the surgical wards were above the medical floor. The south medical wing was the male ward. It had about twenty-five beds, four in a convalescent porch a long way from the nursing station, which was a bench-like desk at one end of the ward. One bed in a private room near the nursing station was reserved for the sickest patient, the one who often caused the most noise and disruption. There were ten beds on each side of a large open room like a banquet hall. If you have visited, or seen pictures of the fifteenth-century Hospices de Beaune in France, or the nineteenth-century hospitals in London, you have a good idea of what it was like. The north wing for women was a mirror image of the men's wing. The spaces were sunny, open, and communal. Privacy was limited to one central treatment room for the floor and a few cloth-covered screens that we moved around as needed. The beds of the sickest patients were wheeled close to the nurses' station where they could receive more attention, especially at night.

Our first task in the morning was to draw blood for lab tests scheduled that day. This was before disposable needles, and recycled needles eventually became dull. It was impossible to tell which were the dull ones until they were tried on a patient. Sometimes the box for sharpening was nearly full after our "blood rounds."

Next we made rounds on each patient with a more seasoned first-year resident. The intern summarized the case and what was new in the last day or two. We were preparing for an attending physician who usually came three days a week to review our progress. The nursing staff was attentive and well trained; the attending-physician teachers were engaged and kept us out of major trouble; and the patients and families were appreciative and generally well behaved.

But all did not go smoothly. Admissions seemed to come in bunches. Night call could be busy all night, and our responsibilities seemed to escalate each day. Admissions from the emergency department arrived without much information. The ER functioned mostly as a triage center. If patients were breathing, had a blood pressure, and were judged sick enough to be hospitalized, they came directly to the medical-floor treatment room. These were the days before cardiac monitors, blood-gases, stat-blood tests, dependable breathing tubes, and mechanical ventilators. Cardiac resuscitation was done in the treatment room. One night we had two resuscitations happening at the same time.

The days and nights I spent on the medical wards solidified my interest in internal medicine. Pneumonia, asthma, diabetes, heart failure, thyroid, liver, and kidney disease were intellectually challenging for a new physician, and there were therapies that truly helped most of our patients. I began to make plans to apply for an internal-medicine residency at the Minneapolis Veterans Administration Hospital. When we rotated to the orthopedic ward, I inherited a patient with a fractured femur who had been in traction for several weeks. In reviewing her record, I noticed an abnormal admission chest X-ray report. She had been given some antibiotics, but was still coughing and had not had any follow-up. The senior orthopedic resident said, "You want to be an internist, you figure out what she has."

When follow-up X-rays showed the upper lung shadow to be unchanged, I put my medical-ward experience to work and ordered sputum cultures, skin tests, and blood work. The next day I received an emergency page from the microbiology lab. They had found "red snappers" in her sputum. "Red snappers" was our expression for acid-fast-staining bacteria, a presumptive sign of active tuberculosis. The orthopedic wards were laid out similar to the medical and surgical wards in big open spaces with about twenty beds lined up along the outside walls. For two weeks our patient had been breathing, coughing, and spitting from an active case of tuberculosis, thus exposing over one hundred people to a difficult-to-treat, life-threatening infection.

The TB-surveillance team went to work, and my patient was isolated. Interviews, X-rays, and skin tests were ordered for patients on the ward. Patient and staff lists were generated, and calls went out to staff workers, discharged patients, and their families. Home visits were made. I never did find out how many total contacts there were or how many new cases of tuberculosis were identified from this patient. I had a Mantoux skin test applied that after forty-eight to seventy-two hours was negative. Since the test was only a few weeks after my exposure, another test needed to be applied in three months. The next test was positive. Now what?

One of Minneapolis's prominent TB specialists was Dr. Sumner Cohen. I brought my chest X-ray to his downtown office. He agreed that it was normal, but since I had a definite skin-test conversion after exposure, he recommended a year on a drug called Isoniazid. Isoniazid was produced in the early 1950s for treating active tuberculosis, but it was just beginning to be used to prevent active disease. Its individual side effects were not well understood because it was usually used in combination with several other drugs. I took the drug for over a year, had trouble remembering my phone number, and only later found out memory issues became a common complication in single-drug Isoniazid therapy. Drug-induced hepatitis was unrecognized at the time, and I did not get peripheral neuritis, the other major drug complication.

Forty-eight years later, a chest CT scan for acute pleurisy revealed the top of both my lungs had scars and a calcified lymph node in a pattern classic for old healed tuberculosis. I had had an active case of tuberculosis that was only recognized by my Mantoux-test conversion.

The surgery wards were less intellectually stimulating but definitely more acutely challenging. Most patients were treated with one sort of dressing or another. Burns were the worst, elective surgery the best. One night an eighteen-year-old store clerk arrived with a gunshot wound to his chest. The emergency room quickly triaged him to the surgical-treatment room as I and the junior surgical resident arrived. The patient was alert, talking, and in minimal pain. An accompanying chest X-ray showed fluid and air in his left chest. While the resident put in a chest tube, I tried to start an IV. These were the days of dull needles and before central catheters were used for venous access. As blood and air came out of his new chest tube, his blood pressure fell and his veins collapsed. "Do a cutdown," yelled the resident. I retrieved a venous-cutdown kit, found the biggest arm vein I could, opened the skin, isolated a vein, threaded in a catheter, and secured it with a strong suture. By that time he had no blood pressure, was no longer awake, and universal-donor blood had arrived. I began pumping air into the glass transfusion bottle, careful not to allow any air to be injected intravenously. This was to be my job for the next hour.

Blood kept coming from the chest tubes (two had been placed by now), his blood pressure had risen to eighty over zero, and the chief surgical resident had arrived. He had alerted the operating room on his drive to the hospital. He took one look at the situation and said, "Let's go."

We rode up the elevator as I pumped unit after unit of blood, some of which was now matched to the patient. The operating room was readied, but the usual hand scrubbing and patient-skin preparation were truncated. Drapes were thrown over the field, the patient was intubated, anesthesia was initiated, and a left chest incision was begun.

All this while, it was my job as the lowest in the surgical hierarchy to keep pumping blood without injecting any air (by this time he had two cutdowns). Anesthesia announced, "Blood pressure eighty over zero."

As the chest was opened, Frank Johnson, the attending chest surgeon, arrived and asked, "What do you have?" to which the chief resident responded, "I don't know. Left chest gunshot wound with pneumothorax and bleeding we can't stop."

Another no-scrub, quickly gowned surgeon joined the team. By now all the drapes were soaked, and most of the floor was covered with blood. There was no obtainable blood pressure, and Dr. Johnson began calling for suction and clamps. "Get more light in the apex [the very top of the chest cavity under the clavicle]! Now suction up there, I can see the bleeder, but I can't reach it. What's the longest clamp you have?" The nurse replied, "You have all the clamps in the surgical pack."

"Can you get me a cervical clamp?" A long cervical clamp from a gynecology pack was produced to clamp the artery. The patient's chest was suctioned out, and the bleeding stopped. Soon the blood pressure rose to near normal, and I stopped pumping. When the operating room began to calm down, the chief resident who couldn't see the bleeding site any clearer than the rest of us asked, "What artery was bleeding?" Dr. Johnson replied, "I don't know, but I am going to tie it off."

The next day the young patient was sitting up in his bed having breakfast. He looked familiar to me. I asked him where he was when he was shot. He said on Thirty-Third and Nicollet Avenue. That was just two blocks from our apartment. He was a clerk in our grocery store! Another patient with an abdominal gunshot wound was admitted a few weeks later. This was less dramatic, but his recovery was much longer. He owned another grocery store that was one block from our house!

Another patient in his twenties tried to kill himself by discharging a pistol under his chin. He succeeded in blowing off his jaw, most of his face, and both eyes. He angled the gun a little too far forward and missed his brain. The surgeons contemplated a repair, but the patient wanted to finish the job he had started. He was placed on the open surgical ward, and in spite of suicide precautions, one night he was found dead in bed. He must have plugged his tracheostomy with his finger and quietly suffocated.

Life changed as 1964 approached. One day, as I walked into the staff-physicians' lounge, the television was on, and everyone was quiet. President Kennedy had been shot in Dallas. As we watched transfixed to the screen for the next few hours, we learned he had died. Later that day Lyndon B. Johnson was sworn in as president. That day, November 22, 1963, and the funeral weekend to follow will be a lifelong memory of shared national grief and reflection.

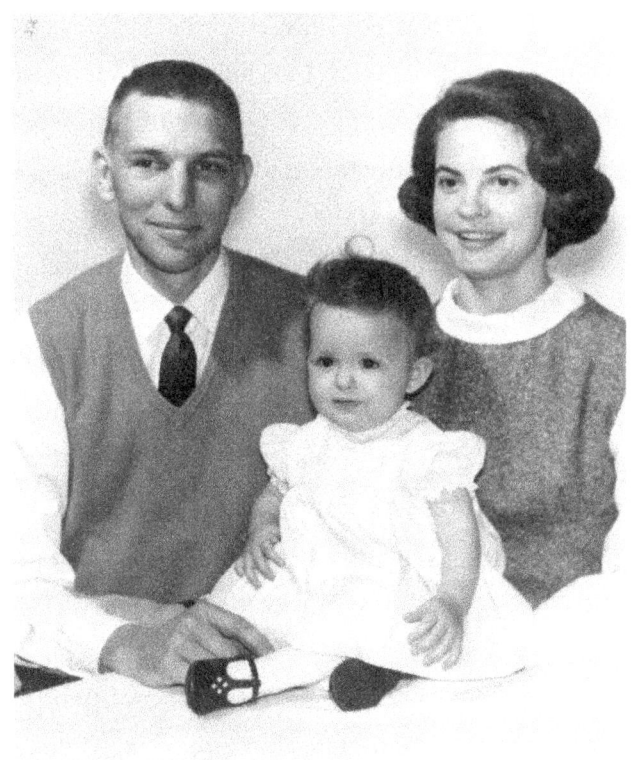

New parents, December 1964

More life changes were to come. Gail and I had our first child two days before Christmas. We thought Marta was the most beautiful child ever born. Gail spent a week in the hospital until I had a chance to take them home. As proud parents, we now had another life to consider. Nights at home were no longer restful. Marta was one of the last babies to be born at Minneapolis General Hospital, as the name would soon be changed.

On January 1, 1964, Hennepin County assumed responsibility for acute trauma and emergency medicine for the western metro area. Minneapolis General Hospital was renamed Hennepin County General Hospital and later Hennepin County Medical Center (HCMC). An intern's salary went from $150 to $310 a month. The odd number was explained: parking, formerly free, now cost $10 a month. When warmer weather came, I started riding my bike and pocketed the $10.

Other rotations came and went. I performed about thirty deliveries on obstetrics; I learned to look in eyes with a slit lamp; I had a rotation on the contagion ward (mostly tuberculosis patients); and I learned to examine noses, throats, and ears.

The big show occurred in the skin clinic. The weekly clinic started at 1:00 p.m. Dr. Layman and his partner would arrive after we had all the patients lined up and gowned. About fifteen residents, interns, and students would sit in close bleacher-like rows. (Visual inspection is everything in dermatology.) The two private-practice attending physicians would arrive from the Minneapolis Club after a lunch that we surmised included more than one adult beverage — these were the days of the two-martini business lunch. One of us interns was charged with writing prescriptions, which meant that we needed to get there early to presign, date, and anticipate the treatment recommendation. When the clinic started, up to forty patients in the lineup would be through in less than an hour.

The patients waiting in the hallway would be called in one by one.

"Take off your gown," Dr Layman would say. "Show us your lesion." The patients were reluctant to bare themselves in front of all the white-coated doctors and students. They were invariably flummoxed and embarrassed, which seemed to delight the flushed-faced doctors. A diagnosis would be barked out. The prescription was usually 1 percent HC and AB, which meant 1 percent hydrocortisone and absorbent base, a greasy ointment that most patients detested. By the time the intern had completed a prepared prescription and the patient had found their gown, the next patient was bare in front of the group. Anyone who needed a biopsy was set aside for the dermatology residents to treat later that afternoon with us interns assisting. In less than an hour a new intern would see the majority of skin diseases prevalent in Minneapolis at that time.

I had more memorable experiences from my rotation in the emergency department. Three of us and a surgical resident managed the doctoring in the department for a four-week period. When needed, we rode with the ambulance on its runs. This was not standard procedure around the country, but was thought to be one of the hospital's benefits for first-year doctors.

I am unsure of the ambulance driver's name. I think it was Alan, but we called him "Big Al." He was a no-nonsense, slightly gruff, large, loveable guy. He had been around the hospital for years and always seemed to make the runs interesting. Whenever I had a chance, I would go with him. Big Al would come into the emergency room and say, "I need a doc." Whoever was free would saddle up with him in front of one of three hearse-like ambulances. There was a stretcher in back, an oxygen tank, a blood-pressure cuff, and not much else. I would ask where we were going and what the call was about: a child hit by a car and unconscious, a suspected stroke, a heart attack, someone with trouble breathing?

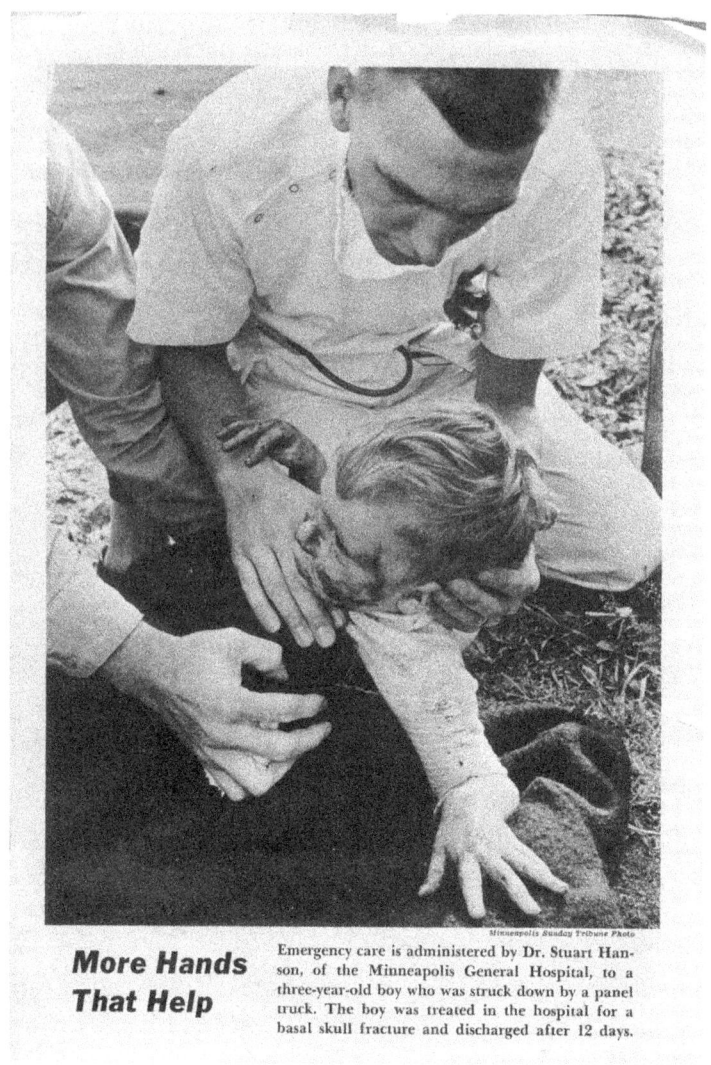

Ambulance doctor, 1963
Reprinted with permission of the Minneapolis Star Tribune

One day I answered his call, and on the ride he said, "One of our psych patients is holding a hostage with a gun." When we arrived at the scene with sirens wailing, four police cars were surrounding a two-story house. About ten policemen were crouched behind the cars with guns drawn. The police captain came over quickly to frame the situation. A male, a person who was known to our psych unit, was holding a female on the second floor and threatening to kill them both if the police came any closer. "Doc, we want you to go up there and get the gun from him." This was definitely a new experience for me. I looked at Big Al, and his eyes said "no way." We begged off and said we would return when he no longer had a gun. Somehow the standoff ended, and a few hours later the police brought the man to the hospital for another admission to the psych ward, a workup by another intern, thus repeating an all-too-frequent cycle.

Another call came in one night. I jumped in the ambulance and was whisked to a deep hole in the ground. An underground worker had been hit by a wall breakout in a sewer tunnel and had a possible broken leg and other injuries. The foreman was ready to lower me in a cage down the shaft to bring him to the surface. When I looked down, I could not see the bottom. I looked at Big Al, who caught my trepidation and said, "The doctor's not allowed to go underground. You'll have to bring him up." With a little instruction on how to move his leg and secure him on a wire stretcher, our patient was loaded into the cage, returned to the surface, and we delivered him to the orthopedists.

One story stands out from all the others. We were not allowed to pick up anyone in the ambulance who was conscious and refused to be treated. A court order was possible in extreme circumstances but rarely used. One night we went on a call to a tenement apartment near the hospital to attend to "a man bleeding and passing out." We arrived to find him lying in bed in a dark room in a pool of clotted blood. He had what looked like chewing tobacco plastered all around his chin. He was alert, but his speech was slurred, and he appeared to be inebriated. I removed the material around his chin to reveal a small laceration about an inch long with pulsating, bright red blood squirting back at me. I applied a pressure dressing, gave him a quick heart, lung, and belly exam. His blood pressure was slightly low and his pulse rapid. When

I sat him up to listen to the back of his lungs, his eyes rolled back. He looked as if he was starting a seizure and he become unconscious. When we laid him back down, he quickly regained consciousness, and I told him he needed to come to the hospital. To our surprise, he adamantly refused. I tried to explain the gravity of the situation and that an adequate repair of his laceration was not possible in the dimly lit, blood-soaked room. He again refused with more vigor than the first time. Only then did I notice on the floor in a dark corner behind me, that a woman who was equally intoxicated, was chewing more tobacco to apply to his wound. She tried to convince him, but we could not change the bleeder's mind. I went to a phone in a hallway to call the ER resident to see if a court order was possible. I distinctly remember cockroaches crawling the walls by the phone.

But no court order was going to be issued or even requested that night. What to do? I asked Big Al, "Can we bring him in if he passes out again?" He agreed we would be on "solid ambulance guidelines" if that happened.

I said, "I think we need to sit him up again." When we did, the patient passed out, and we loaded him onto the stretcher. By the time he woke up, we had him in the ambulance on our way to the hospital. Four units of blood, a few well-placed sutures, a night's sleep, and a good breakfast put him on his way the next day. He did not return again that year.

Did we interns get a well-rounded, liberal, medical education that year? Did we learn to take responsibility and do the best we could for the patients who came under our care? Did we come away feeling we had made a good choice of career? Most of us could answer yes to these questions. My rarely seen roommate was licensed and took a position as a general practitioner in a small western Minnesota town for $2,000 a month, guaranteed. Many decades later he was convicted of molesting young boys in his office and sentenced to a long term in federal prison.

THE GENERAL

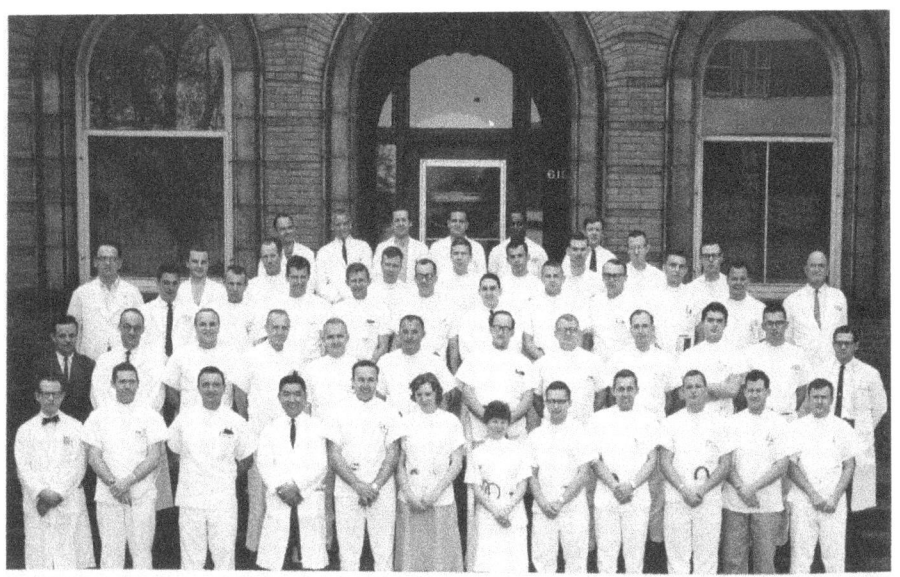

*Hennepin County General Hospital intern and resident staff, 1964
I am in the third row, third from the right.*

(Unable to identify photogtapher or copyright.)

CHAPTER THIRTEEN

Our Introduction to Asia

Any male entering the medical field as a physician in the 1960s was aware of the "doctors' draft." Two years of compulsory government service were part of your career plan if you wanted to be a physician, dentist, or veterinarian. In order to avoid being conscripted into an unwanted military service, I signed up for the Navy's Ensign 1915 program as a second-year medical student at Dartmouth. Service longevity started when you were accepted into the program. By the time I was inducted in August 1965, I had been an inactive-duty ensign for four years. I was able to choose my branch of service and had longevity, which added to my active-duty pay grade. We then began three years of living in Japan. I spent one year in and out of the South China Sea as the Vietnam War was ramping up. It was a life-changing experience of war, submersion into an Asian culture, and tending our growing family overseas.

As my internship was coming to a close, I wanted to delay active duty to complete specialty training. I applied for deferment through what was called the Berry Plan. In 1964 our country's involvement in Southeast Asia was progressing along uncertain lines. That meant deferments for specialty training were limited. I received a one-year reprieve and started an internal-medicine residence at the Minneapolis VA Hospital and the University of Minnesota. By March 1965, I knew my time had come. A night attack on a U.S. ship in the Tonkin Gulf off Vietnam, which later was proven to be fabricated, prompted a Congressional resolution. President Lyndon B. Johnson and Congress led us into another land war in Asia. My deferment was not extended.

I expected to receive my notice for active military duty. Gail was pregnant with our second child due in early July, just at the time I was to start service in the U.S. Navy as a general medical officer. The timing was not ideal. We were interested in traveling to another part of the world like Europe, but had not considered Asia, especially with an armed conflict brewing.

The year 1965 was the beginning of a tumultuous period in U.S. history. A buildup of military forces in Southeast Asia was occurring. The first U.S. Marines did eventually land at Chu Lai, Vietnam, in May, initiating a land invasion in Asia, the first since Korea in the 1950s.

We did have some choices. I looked into conscientious-objector status for national service and found I was not registered and therefore not eligible at this late date. We could leave the country with no guarantee of return, or I could refuse Naval induction, be charged with desertion, and go to federal prison for up to five years. There was no guarantee I would have a medical license on release. And so; we decided to deal with the uncertainty of a military assignment.

I got on the phone with the U.S. Naval Bureau of Personnel. After several calls, I was transferred to a physician, Captain Lonergan, in the Pentagon. I told him we wanted an assignment in Europe. He said, "No way." He proposed several options with the Marines: Camp Pendleton near San Diego, Twenty-Nine Palms in the California desert, and China Lake Naval Air Station (another desert location). All were Marine assignments, which might be headed to Southeast Asia for a year. I said, "What else do you have?" By now he must have begun losing patience with this neophyte Naval Reservist. He tried Oakland, California, an ammunition center. When I asked what the duty was like, he mumbled something I couldn't understand. When I asked him to repeat, he said, "Doctor, it's D-U-L-L, dull."

The conversation had gone on too long, and I could tell it was time to make a decision. So I said, "What do you have in Japan that doesn't require a three-year commitment?" That's when he brought up a landing-ship-squadron medical-officer assignment home-ported in Japan. He didn't know what I'd be doing — it would be at least a year of sea duty, then a possible transfer to a naval hospital somewhere for the second year. He could make no promises, and my assignment would be made at least thirty days before I had to report. And, yes, I could bring my family.

With time running out, I said I would like the Japan assignment, and our conversation was over. Months went by. We were anxious to learn where we were going and how we were going to manage a household move with a new baby and Marta, our 1½-year-old daughter. When the orders came, they were in "Navy speak." It read "Report to Comlanshipron9," which took days to decipher. The Naval Air Station in Minneapolis studied the communication and decided it meant, "Report to the commanding officer of landing ships squadron nine," which I learned was home-ported in Yokosuka, Japan. I would be getting my basic introduction to the Navy at an amphibious base in Coronado, California, across the bay from San Diego. That was the first time I had heard of Yokosuka.

Gail was enthusiastic about going to Japan. So was I, but I was less enthusiastic about a year or more at sea. Then we had Pedro Gonzales Vivian Emanuel to consider — that was the name we used to acknowledge our incubating child — who was a couple of months from his (or her) expected birth.

About the first of July, a week before Gail was due to deliver, she noted a large lump in one breast. She saw her obstetrician who immediately contacted a surgeon. They both agreed this development could be serious, and surgery was scheduled for July 3.

In those days breast cancer was treated with a radical mastectomy. Biopsies were not taken before surgery then. The doctor simply scheduled surgery as though a total mastectomy would be performed. The patient was anesthetized not knowing what would be done. The procedure might take an hour or up to four hours, depending on what the surgeon found. We would not accept this approach as a community standard of practice now. Mammograms, magnetic-resonance imaging (MRI), ultrasound, needle biopsies, and days or even weeks of sifting through statistical data and treatment options are currently the norm. And we had Pedro to consider.

I was relieved when the surgeon came to the waiting room after an hour and reported that Gail had a benign milk cyst and was in the recovery room. This was what I expected and hoped for. Little did I know that the biggest event of the day was yet to come.

I met Gail in her room on the surgical floor, and we sat together enjoying our relief. When Gail went to sleep in the evening, I went home to catch up with our daughter and get some sleep.

Soon Gail called me back to the hospital. She had started having contractions, and her roommate called the nurses, saying, "Get this woman out of here!"

Gail was moved to the obstetrical ward. Her labor had begun as soon as the surgical sedation wore off. The surgical nurses did not want to deliver a newborn on their floor.

Gail's labor was much shorter than the twenty-eight hours with Marta. When Pedro presented himself as a healthy boy, we rejoiced, modified his in-utero name to Peter, and began preparing ourselves for the move to Japan. We were about to have the experience of a lifetime.

OUR INTRODUCTION TO ASIA

Packers came to collect what secondhand furniture and household items we had accumulated in two years of marriage. Three and a half weeks after Peter was born, we gave up our lower duplex apartment and turned over some of our life possessions to the Navy for transport to Japan and some for safe storage. Our lives were becoming a government commodity. We were told our orders allowed concurrent travel, which meant that all four of us could travel together. What we didn't know was that children under two years did not rate a seat (we had two). They were to occupy an adult's lap.

August came and I left for two weeks of naval assimilation in Coronado, California. Gail stayed at her parents' home in Minneapolis to manage our growing family. The newborn wouldn't need any immunizations, but Gail and Marta, our eighteen-month old, would. A few days before they were to fly to San Francisco, where we were to meet for our flight to Japan, they had their shots. Marta reacted with a high fever. Gail's parents had left town, so my mother was enlisted to bathe Marta in cold water all night to reduce the fever while Gail dealt with Peter.

A few days later Gail started for San Francisco. Checking in at the airport in Minneapolis, she discovered that not only had the Navy denied her a second seat for the three of them, but the bulkhead seat requested for the baby basket wasn't available either. Gail had to fly with two children under two on her lap. Then she had to change planes in Denver. When I met them at the San Francisco airport, Gail was glad to give me Marta and the bags as she held Peter, and we headed to a friend's house for the night.

Our U.S. departure site was Travis Air Force Base north of San Francisco. When we arrived, we found there was only one seat for Lieutenant Hanson. My lap was not big enough for three others, and I began to seek options. I asked for the plane's manifest. My name was the sole Hanson on the list. I was told to send my family back to Minneapolis, to find housing in Japan, and then to "bring them over."

By this time I had some experience with military procedures. I asked for the officer in charge. When an Air Force captain appeared — the equivalent rank to me, a Navy lieutenant — I explained our situation and produced my orders. He agreed concurrent travel was authorized, but said the plane was fully booked. I asked for the manifest again and looked for the two lowest-ranking personnel. I asked to have those seats. He reluctantly agreed and bumped the unfortunate cadets. Now we had three seats for the four of us — luxury compared to Gail's earlier experience.

The flight to Tachikawa airport outside of Tokyo was uneventful. Our children mostly ate and slept. Gail and I speculated on what our new life would bring. We were met by our physician host for a two-hour drive to Yokosuka. We collapsed onto the rice-straw mats in a Japanese-style hotel room. This was to be our home for the next week while I reported for duty, and we looked for permanent housing.

When I reported to Yokusuka Naval Base, I learned that the squadron commodore, my commanding officer, was out to sea. One of the LST ship captains seemed to know I was coming, and I started to meet the Navy medical corpsmen I would be supervising.

Gail and I were not authorized for Naval-base housing and needed to live off the base, but, we had to consider our two young children. When we were taken to a small two-story house set among a series of terraced rice paddies, we looked at each other and questioned whether this was a good idea, since I would be at sea for long periods. The owner said, "Yakosan lives nearby. She was the maid for the previous renter. I know she is available." After glancing at each other, we said, "Let's go for it." Thus began three years of a new life in Japan for us and our children.

OUR INTRODUCTION TO ASIA

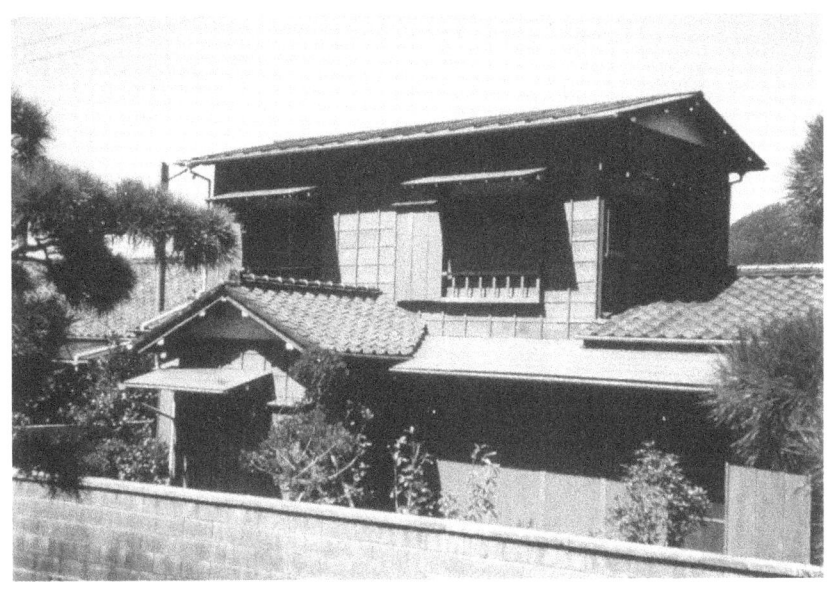

Front of 1150 Shimoyama Guchi, Hayama, Japan

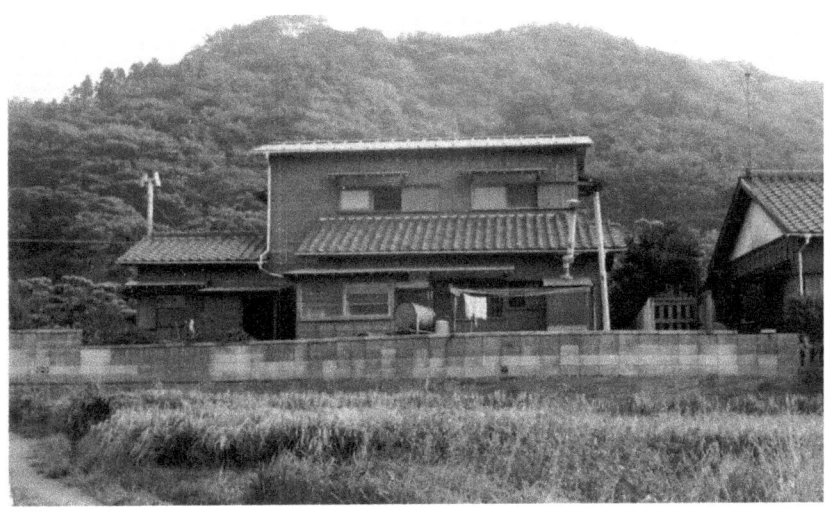

Rear of our house among local rice paddies

CHAPTER FOURTEEN

War Zone

Naval ships that move combat tanks and other vehicles are called "Landing Ship Tanks" or LSTs. They were the main transporters of vehicles and supporting troops in World War Two. After a beachhead has been secured, these ships open their large bow doors, sail directly onto a beach, drop a ramp, and discharge vehicles and personnel. LSTs were to become my home away from home for a year after I reported for active duty in August 1965. For a young physician whose medical education was largely in laboratories and hospitals treating sick people, it would be a year of applying my medical knowledge to military operations that used healthy personnel. I would be the medical officer for eight LSTs home-ported in Yokosuka, Japan. Yokosuka had been the Japanese Fleet Headquarters until it was surrendered to the United States in 1945. The ships and men were healthy when I reported for duty, but that was about to change.

My first voyage was aboard the Windom County — all LSTs are named after U.S. counties. It was a beautiful day as we came out of Tokyo Bay and headed west. We were going to practice a beach landing near the foot of Mt. Fuji. The sunset with shades of pink, orange, and grey was beautiful. The sunrise the next morning on Mt. Fuji, the iconic Japanese mountain, was spectacular. The beach landing went well, and that night we headed for Okinawa.

Our orders were secret, but we suspected we would be transporting Marines and their equipment from Okinawa to Vietnam through the South China Sea. I was surprised that the officers and enlisted men were anxious to get to a battlefield. Healthy young men were anxious to go into harm's way, and my job would be to patch them up, if they survived. I had been trained to prevent disease and injury. Now I had to prepare for the worst.

LSTs have flat bottoms that are needed for beach landings. But at sea their ride can be rough. Their roll from side to side was severe even in modest seas. They also bent slightly in the middle as they rode over an oncoming wave rather than cut through it as most ships do. This led to an up-and-down ship vibration called "stumping." An LST that was rolling, pitching, and stumping aggravated even experienced sailors' stomachs.

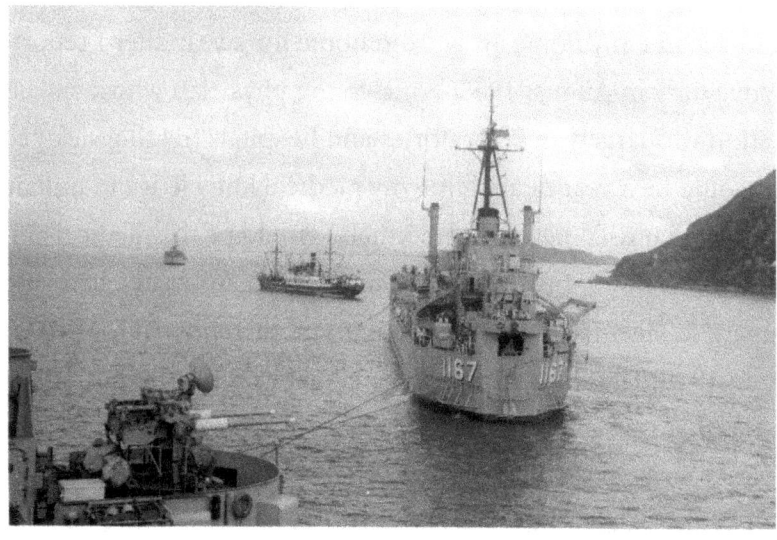

Stern view of an LST built after WW II

WAR ZONE

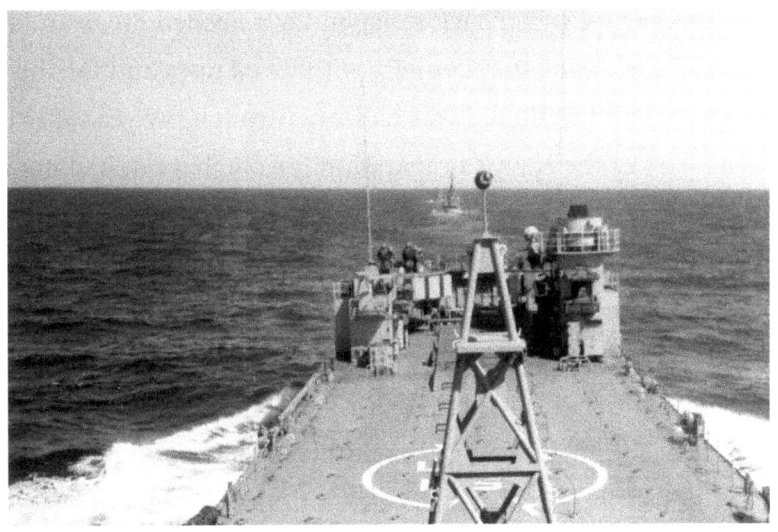

View from the command bridge toward an LST bow

Our first load of vehicles and Marines from Okinawa was landed on a beach at Chu Lai, where the Marines had made their first landing in May. I visited the field of tents and muddy paths that made up the camp. The medical officers were proud of their surgical and infirmary tents. I was glad to get back to my beached ship.

Thus began our routine for the next five months. We would load Marines and their vehicles in Naha, Okinawa, and deliver them to a beach along the South Vietnam coast — Da Nang, Quy Nhon (qui non), Tuy Hoa (tooy wah), Nha Trang (nah trang), Cam Ranh (cam rawn) Bay, Phan Thiet (fan thiet), and Vung Tau (vung tao). I learned to read tide-tables and beach hydrography, and was moved from one ship to another to assist new commanding officers making their first beach landings. All of the landings were unopposed except for an occasional ship-side explosion that always came at night. No ships were damaged, and some of us thought the explosions may have been friendly grenades set off to earn the crew's hostle-fire pay for the month.

In December we sailed back to Japan for a needed break and the holidays. It was a time to reconnect with loved ones and for ships to be repaired and refitted. I was halfway through my year at sea. I had been part of the Navy's preparation for combat but had not seen much action.

Most of our eight-ship LST squadron headed out of Tokyo Bay in early 1966 not knowing what our next assignment would be. Most of the ships' crews were surprised we were going to Pusan, Korea. The U.S. Marines had landed in South Vietnam, and now the Korean Marines were joining the fight. The flotilla included about twenty-five ships including personnel carriers (APAs), landing ships dock (LSDs), a command cruiser, destroyer escorts, and our LSTs. This impressive armada sailed through the Taiwan Straits close to mainland China and though the South China Sea to Vietnam. These Korean Marines were the famed Tiger Division who later became known as fierce fighters who took few prisoners.

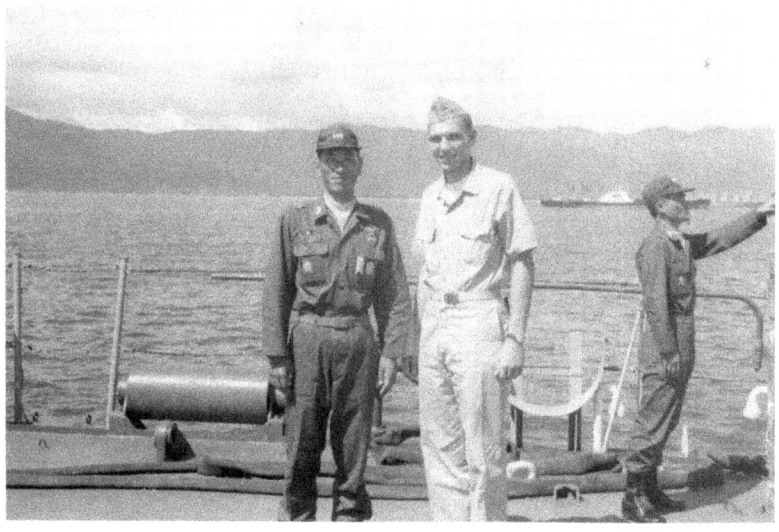

The Korean Tiger Division commander and me en route to Nha Trang, Vietnam

When LSTs landed with their bows nosed into the beach, their greatest threat was broaching — moving sideways from the currents and tides and becoming parallel to the beach, thus making it impossible to get off. Broaching was prevented by dropping a stern anchor long before hitting the beach. Tension on the anchor cable kept the ship perpendicular to the shore.

One day we received a message that one of our LSTs had broached at Tuy Hoa. My ship was dispatched to the scene. The ship's crew was still aboard, but the ship had no power. Eventually it took two large sea tugboats to extract it. The ship had listed to one side, could not make fresh water, and could only power an auxiliary generator. The health concerns for the crew led my commodore to assign me to accompany the towed ship back to Japan. During the slow-towed trip back to Japan for repairs, I asked my medical corpsman how the ship broached after its landing. He was reluctant at first, but eventually shared the crew's opinion that the captain had not dropped the stern anchor in time to keep the ship perpendicular to the shore. When the tide came, resulting currents had swung the ship's stern and broached the ship.

In 1966 the land war in Vietnam was heating up. The Viet Cong (VC), who were communist insurgents fighting for South Vietnam independence, were firing recoil-less rifles at merchant ships sailing up the rivers to Saigon. A multiservice operation, called Starlight, was initiated to root out the VC who were dug into tunnels throughout the area. I was assigned to the LST designated to be the command ship sitting in the Soai Rap River alongside a small village.

The surrounding area had been defoliated with Agent Orange (a product containing toxic dioxins). Dive bombers spent days targeting tunnel entrances. Artillery batteries in the village fired repeatedly toward out-of-view targets. Navy bombers dropped napalm tanks on in-view villages. We had warning when highflying, unseen B-52 bombers were scheduled to drop their saturation bomb loads. At night, our

LST and other smaller river boats bombarded the shores with gun and rocket fire. The available ordinance of the U.S. Military was on display.

After days and nights of exploding ordinance, the captain of our ship became distressed to the point he couldn't function. There have been various names used for battle fatigue — shell shock and more recently post traumatic stress disorder (PTSD). He knew he was disabled when his fellow officers came to me, but it was my job to evaluate him and make a recommendation to my commanding officer. The commodore was on another ship away from the action, and he instructed me to do what I thought was needed and right. The ship's other officers supported my decision to relieve the captain. I had to escort him to a medical facility. The ship's captain, carrying his belongings, and I climbed into a small boat and were driven to shore. All nearby medical facilities were inundated with wounded and had no capacity to help us. We commandeered rides and flights to Saigon. The general commanding the army hospital in Saigon was astounded at the prospects of relieving a Naval ship's captain for a mental breakdown. It would be the end of the captain's career. Fortunately for both the general and me, our patient agreed with the transfer. I then had to retrace my route back to the battleground, but I had solved a problem that was inhibiting our part of the operation.

I was relieved to receive orders to report to the naval hospital in Yokosuka in July of 1966. My year of sea duty had put me in positions for which I had little preparation. I had had direct war experiences and I had survived physically. I had expanded my knowledge of war and the men who fight them. I returned to practice medicine in more familiar surroundings caring for the sick and injured evacuated from the battlefields. I avoided ribbons or awards while serving and was relieved to be separated from active duty in 1968. When I finally received a full discharge in 1969, I was surprised to see two bronze star awards listed in my record. I never looked up why. They had some ceremonies but I never went. I didn't think award giving was appropriate in a time of war.

CHAPTER FIFTEEN

Life on the Beach

When Gail and I married in 1963, we did not plan on moving to a field of rice paddies in Japan. We knew I was obligated for two years of military service sometime, but that was off in the future. But in 1965 the future had arrived, and we had two children under two to consider. I was assigned to a landing-ship squadron of tank-transport ships homeported in Yokosuka, Japan.

We were excited about living in a foreign country, but naïve about the effort and risk we were taking. Once in Japan, we found a house to our liking and began building a new life. Looking back we're still not sure how we managed and sometimes doubt that we could do it again. However, it became one of the life-changing events that defined our values, beliefs, and actions.

We rented a house at 1150 Shimoyama Guchi, near Sagami Bay and the village of Hayama. It became our home for two and a half years. Our daughter, Marta, was twenty months old and our son, Peter, was just six weeks.

Our street started at a bay of the Pacific Ocean called Sagami Wan—wan being the Japanese word for bay. Looking at a map of Japan, it is the first bay west of Tokyo Bay where the Yokosuka Naval Base was located. The two bays are separated by a low mountain range forming a peninsula. The Emperor of Japan at the time, Hirohito, had a summer palace on Sagami Wan at the end of our street. Our house was about halfway up the valley of Shimoyama, which means "shining mountain." Guchi is the Japanese word for valley. A small stream coming off the mountain flowed a short ways from the winding road in front of our house. As we walked up our street's gentle incline, the houses became more scattered. Rice paddies filled in the gaps, and gave us the sense of living among tiers of small, hand-tilled, farm fields. All the houses were small, made of wood, and roofed with tile. Most had tiny walled-in yards and plantings with something blooming year-round.

Our house had two stories, which was unusual as most were single-storied. The living rooms of the one-storied houses became sleeping rooms by bringing futon bedding from nearby closets and placing them on the tatami-matted floors. A tatami mat was about two inches thick, two and a half feet wide, and five feet long. They were uniform in size all over Japan. They could be fitted to conform to specific room sizes. Living rooms were described by the number of tatami mats they had. An eight-tatami room was always the same size. We had two eight-mat rooms on the first floor. On the second floor, there was an eight-mat master bedroom and a six-mat children's bedroom.

Separate hard-floor rooms for kitchen, dining, and bathing were on the first floor. Each room was heated separately in the winter with portable kerosene heaters. The toilet facilities were international. All cultures were accommodated. There was a single washbasin in a hallway leading to three separate self-contained stalls. The first stall was a urinal. Next came an Asian style straddle-and-squat-type, with a flushable trough. Last in the line of stalls was a Western-type commode.

LIFE ON THE BEACH

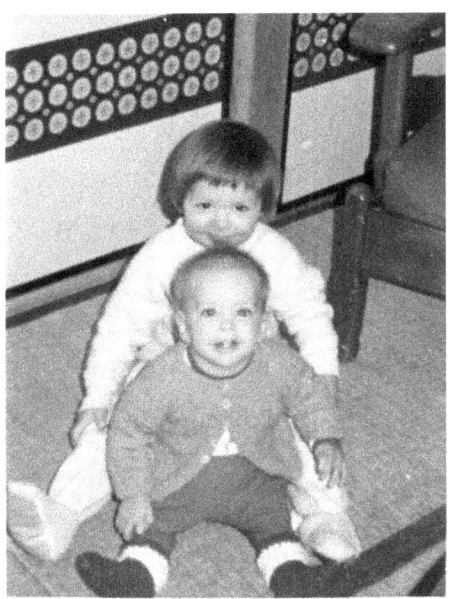

Marta and Peter on our rice straw "tatami" floor mats with paper closet doors in the background

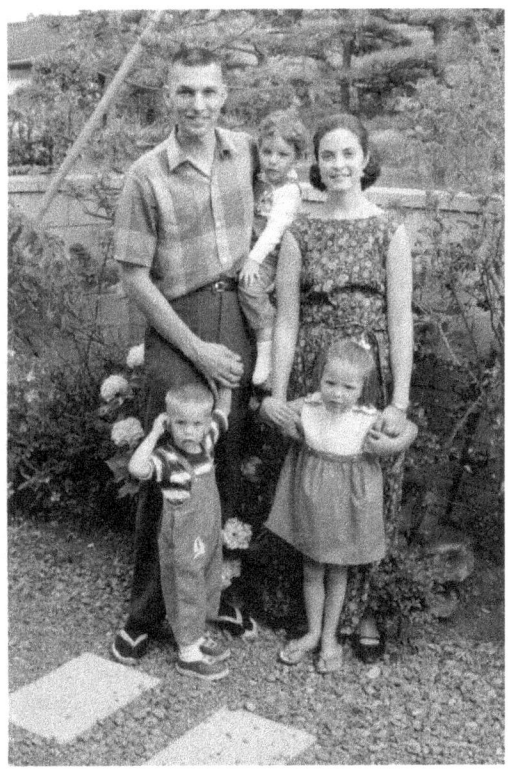

I am holding a friend's child in our enclosed garden, 1967.

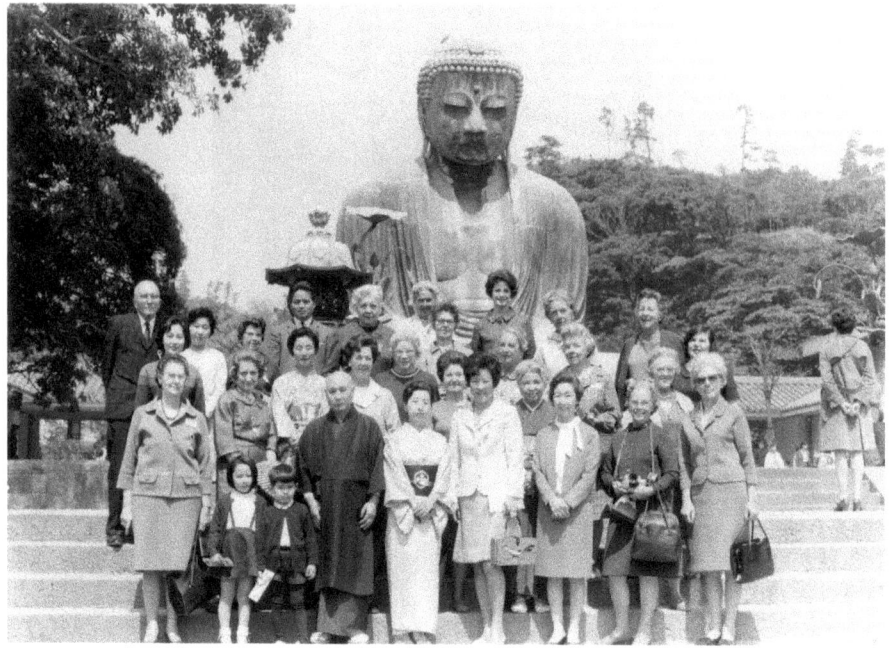

Gail's Yokosuka-Kamakura Cultural Society. She is the tallest in the back row.

This corner of the house had no heat. In the winter the commode could be covered with a thin sheet of ice. Accommodating Americans had its price. The second year we installed a fuel-oil space heater for winters and an air conditioner for summers in the matted living rooms.

We had a maid five days a week, and she doubled as a babysitter anytime we needed evening or weekend childcare. By the time I had completed my year of sea duty, Gail had established herself in the Japanese-American community. She was teaching high-school conversational English in Hiratska, Japan. She belonged to the Yokosuka-Kamakura Cultural Society, and she became accomplished in fish rubbing, flower arranging, brush painting, and the elements of the Japanese tea ceremony.

LIFE ON THE BEACH

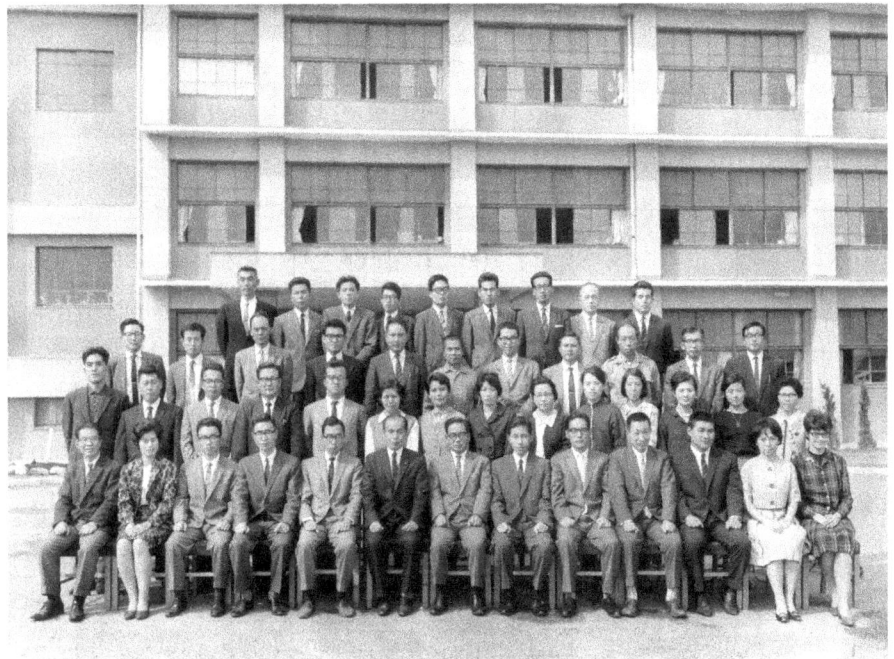

Hiratska high-school teachers, 1967. Gail is in the first row, far right.

After my year at sea, I had a lot of catching up to do. I watched the farmers walking to their fields with hand implements, wading and digging in the flooded paddies, hand-planting rice shoots (done only by fertile women), harvesting after drying the fields at season's end, and carrying the produce on their backs to their homes.

I watched the Tokyo businessmen walking down our dirt road to the bus in the morning and back in the evening. We got to know a few of them, but mostly we were observers of the ebb and flow of daily life. We enjoyed our lives to the point that we extended our tour for another year to absorb more of the fascinating Asian culture.

When our time in Japan was coming to a close in 1968, we wanted to do some traveling in Asia before we returned to the United States. We moved to the Naval Base at Yokosuka so Marta could attend an English-speaking preschool and hired a maid who could take care of the children while we traveled.

We planned a trip to India in February of 1968. We were due to leave Japan in June and first wanted to explore more of Asia. Then the Tet Offensive, the biggest and most violent of the then three-year war, hit in Vietnam. It started just days before we were to leave Japan on space-available military aircraft. The Army, Air Force, and Marines had canceled all leaves, but the Navy had not. My commanding officer wished I would stay, but said, "Your orders give you twelve days' leave that has not been canceled." I thanked him and quickly left his office before he could change his mind.

Every aircraft going south was full. We were finally seated on a transport going to Okinawa. Once there, we booked a commercial flight to Taiwan, but it was suddenly canceled. The next four flights over the next twenty-four hours were also canceled. Then we learned that the one plane scheduled for all the flights had crashed, and there would be no more flights to Taiwan. We had to alter our plans. Trans World Airlines (TWA) could get us to Hong Kong and eventually to Bangkok. We received sketchy news about the escalating war in Vietnam, which we had to cross to get to Thailand.

The evening flight from Hong Kong to Bangkok was going smoothly. Drinks and dinner were served, and we settled in for the next few hours. Then the captain announced, "We will be going over South Vietnam in the next few minutes. We will be at 30,000 feet, well out of gun range."

That was encouraging. Then he added, "You might want to look out the windows. Those fires you see are burning villages."

Out of the darkness we saw a patchwork of orange on a black background — Halloween colors representing the horror below. We stared for ten minutes, and then we passed over the war zone and were headed to the rest-and-recreation destination of Bangkok. Our experience seems surreal, even after fifty years.

In Bangkok we were able to get space on what was called an "embassy flight" — a flight that diplomatic couriers use between the world's capitals where the United States has diplomatic presence. The view of the Ganges River delta 35,000 feet below is hard to forget. It looked like a web with convoluted, interconnected channels, like the surface of an exposed brain.

Each country in Asia presented us with a new culture. We experienced the contrast between the dignified boulevards, spaciously placed houses, and European architecture of New Delhi and the crowded, congested mass of buildings and crowds of street humanity in Old Delhi. The Taj Mahal, said to be the most beautiful building in the world, did not disappoint us.

On our return, the embassy flights going east had space for us all the way back to Japan. That was the good news. The bad news was that our flight was to be the first to land in Saigon since the Tet Offensive had begun.

The flight from New Delhi to Bangkok was uneventful. The pilot said he was not sure if we would be able to land in Saigon. As we approached, he said the descent was going to be steep because the airport perimeter was not secure. I knew what this meant, but did not tell Gail. Luckily she didn't ask.

I saw the airport below us, but we were too high. Then the pilot said, "We are going to make a sharp turn to the left and descend. It will feel like I've lost control of the plane, and you will feel like your stomach is in your feet."

Since Okinawa we had not had any major travel upsets. That was to end in Saigon. The landing was really tough, and we were relieved to feel the runway. Then we noticed we had taxied to the center of the field and stopped. We disembarked to walk about a quarter mile to the terminal. Gail was in her pastel, light tropical dress and I was in my tropical, short-sleeved, white officer's uniform. We were told the Boeing 727 was a strong target, and it was not safe to move it to the terminal.

Inside the terminal we found personnel busily filling sandbags and piling them along the walls of our waiting room. This went on for an hour in the humid tropical heat. When we were summoned to the plane, I was nervous about leaving the comfort of a protected, sand-bagged space to walk to a plane that was a Viet Cong target.

We returned to the plane and quickly taxied to the end of the runway and took off fast. Gail and I were relieved to be in the air again. The landings in the Philippines, Okinawa, and finally Tokyo brought a memorable day to a close.

We made plans to return to the United States by ship. The military transferred some personnel using the American President Lines. The USS *Polk* was a commercial cruising ship and had all the luxuries of pleasure travel: comfortable staterooms, sitting lounges, a play area for our children with attendants, and first-class meals. We looked forward to a relaxing end to our time in Asia.

On the day of departure our family hosted a going-away party on the ship for the friends we were leaving behind. After the champagne was opened, a loudspeaker announcement blurted, "Lieutenant Arthur Hanson, please report to the gangway."

Now what? Would our departure be delayed? Had I neglected to do something? Were my orders being changed?

When I arrived at the gangway a deck man asked, "Is that your car?" Thirty feet below on the dock was a dark blue, 1962 Oldsmobile station wagon. It was the one we brought from Minnesota and had left in Yokohama to be shipped to San Francisco.

"Yes, that's my car." And with that response, the deck man circled his arm, the ship's boom raised the car, swung it into a hold, and the all-visitors-ashore signal was given. I barely had time to say good-bye to our friends as they rushed off the ship and we sailed away.

The fourteen-day Pacific crossing included a day in Hawaii before we sailed under the Golden Gate Bridge into San Francisco. Here the ship rule of "last on first off" operated well. As the four of us walked off the gangway, our car was unloaded at our feet. We gathered our luggage and drove off to experience life in the United States in 1968. Martin Luther King, Jr. had been assassinated in Memphis. Robert Kennedy's assassination, the Democratic-Convention riots, and multiple city riots were soon to follow.

Our family's years in Japan triggered our fascination for world geography, politics, culture, and natural beauty. All four of us have traveled to remote parts of the world and have developed an appreciation of nature and humanity that we would not have had otherwise. Marta, a Chinese-medical historian, says her interest in Asia came from her early childhood experiences. Peter, a world-sports-medicine physician, has similar feelings. Gail and I have traveled on seven continents and seven seas in the last fifty years.

CHAPTER SIXTEEN

The Road Less Traveled

Taking time away from one's major activities such as education or work is an honored and institutionally embedded tradition. Vacations, holidays, long weekends are part of most workers' lifestyles. Carving out a longer block of time — a month, a quarter, a semester, a year — is more rare, unless you are a university academic, and then it may be more or less a requirement. I began taking a less traditional route in college, and it has made all the difference.

My goals on entering Dartmouth College in 1955 were to get a well-rounded liberal arts education and to play division-one athletics, after which I hoped to attend medical school. I declared premed as a potential major, which meant I had to take a series of chemistry, math, physics, and biological-science courses. There was a two-year language requirement that could be met in one year by taking an intensive French course six mornings a week, plus three afternoon conversation sessions. I signed up.

There wasn't much time for history, literature, or art. One of my "liberal arts" goals was to take a course in geology — termed "rocks" in the Dartmouth student vernacular. I have yet to take a formal "rocks" course.

Dartmouth Medical School provided only the first two years of medical school. But it offered entrance to a class of twenty-four students after three years of college. I was intrigued. My four-year tuition-and-books scholarship would cover the first year of medical school. My sister, Eileen, would soon enter college, and the more independent I was, the more opportunity she might have. There were over 300 premed students in our freshman class in 1955. There were still one hundred of us during our junior year, two and a half years later, when I might apply to start medical school my senior year.

I sent in my application and waited. I was invited for an interview after which I was sure I would be rejected. I was interviewed by a psychiatry professor who mumbled, "If you were going to interview an applicant for medical school, what would you ask them?" I had to ask him to repeat his garbled question before answering.

I listed a set of questions that I thought would be pertinent. Then he mumbled something I again didn't understand. When I asked him to repeat, he clearly said. "Is that all?" I came up with two more questions and stopped. He again said, "Is that all?" When I said yes, he said, "Now interview yourself."

I went through each of the ten questions as I desperately tried to remember what I had said originally. When I stopped, he mumbled something. I again had to ask him what he said. He said, "Is that all?" When I said yes, he said, "That's all," and our interview was over.

I had little hope that my application would be successful. Then on January 2, 1958, a thin letter arrived from the medical-school secretary. In a few sentences it stated that I had been accepted for the class starting in September, if I remitted $100 in the next 10 days. Now I had to make the decision to forgo a senior year pursuing a philosophy-of-religion major and begin medical school. For the time being a liberal arts education would have to wait.

There wasn't much time for the liberating arts during the first two years of medical school. I returned to downhill skiing, resigned from the basketball team, started to smoke a pipe, and attended a Great Issues course required of all seniors. But I felt I had not had the broadening experience of my classmates when we received our bachelor degrees in June 1959. A second year of medical school didn't offer much more than pathology, microbiology, pharmacology, neuropsychiatry, physical diagnosis, and statistics.

As the second year continued, my classmates began making plans to transfer to another school for the remaining two clinical years. One of our classmates, John Remers, was invited by the physiology department to spend the next year in research at Dartmouth. I sought similar opportunities and found a post-sophomore research grant from National Institutes of Health (NIH). The pharmacology department agreed to sponsor me, and my application was approved. I would have a year of modest income, an opportunity to get seriously involved in research, and to audit any course I wanted in the college. I would be off the academic progression of an MD degree and have time to explore the world of research, attend the lectures of revered Dartmouth professors, and travel outside the country. (I have described the "Summer of 1961" in a previous chapter.) The fifteen months between finishing my second year of medical school at Dartmouth and starting my third year at the University of Minnesota were especially rewarding.

Gail and I were married the day after I graduated from the University of Minnesota Medical School in June of 1963. Since I had made an effort to be exposed to a liberal college education, I chose to take a rotating internship to get a broad "liberal" medical education before starting an internal-medicine residency. The Minneapolis General Hospital did not disappoint. The experiences at what we called "The General" gave me a solid foundation for the next fifty years.

When the U.S. Navy interrupted my internal-medicine residency after the first of three years in 1965, Gail and I took our family to Japan where I would be home-ported for a year and then assigned to a hospital for a second year. Gail submerged herself in a new culture, while I made assault landings in Vietnam. We decided to extend our stay in Japan, which allowed us to explore the country and travel to Thailand and India.

Looking back on our Japanese experience, I realize that our family is more aware of the world's diverse populations and its geopolitical alignments. In the 1970s we spent four to six weeks every other year traveling to the East Coast, the West Coast, Canada, Mexico and the Yucatan, Europe, and South America.

In the 1980s we followed our daughter, Marta, to France where she was an exchange student, and to China where she was studying. When our son, Peter, went off to college, we took a three-month sabbatical to visit friends and family in Asia: Pakistan, India, Nepal, Singapore, Malaysia, Indonesia, China, and Japan. In 1989 we made a "roots trip" to Scandinavia visiting Denmark, Norway, Finland, and family in Sweden. Two years later we took a train trip from Berlin to Bejing across Germany, Poland, Russia, Siberia, and Mongolia. In the 2000s Gail and I spent a month in Italy, visited Iceland, and went to Antarctica, our seventh continent.

Where do these times away from our daily activities over five decades leave us now? Marta is a Chinese-medical and East Asian public health historian at Johns Hopkins University and she frequently spends time in France, Germany, Korea, and China. Peter is a family-practice and sports-medicine physician in Nevada who travels with the U.S. world-sports teams and volunteers at the U.S. Olympic Training Center in Colorado as a team physician. In 2015 Gail and I took an around-the-world 108-day cruise from Miami to Miami sailing on six of the seven seas. In 2016 we sailed on the seventh sea through the Arctic Northwest Passage from Anchorage to New York over Canada.

Our family has been fortunate. When we went off the expected path and took some risks, the experience generally was positive and expansive. I kept working to age seventy-five because I liked the work and didn't tire of the stresses of medical practice and its continuous changes. Gail found her passion in quilt making and retired from university teaching twenty years earlier. Our daughter and son are productive adults engaged in the world. So far none of us has burned out in our main professional activity. Taking time out has had a major impact on our lives. I feel it has made us more aware of our common humanity, more willing to commit our time and talents to help others, and maybe, just maybe, we will leave the world a better place when we are finished.

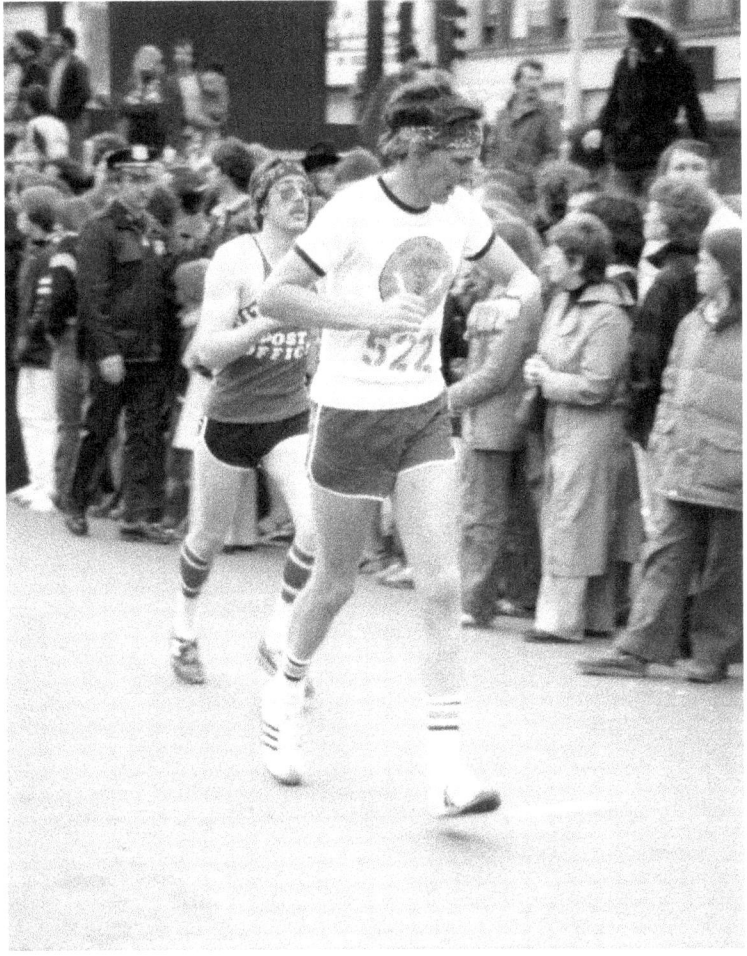

Boston Marathon finish under four hours (3 hrs. 59 min. 59 sec.), 1978

CHAPTER SEVENTEEN

Accidental Trafficking

A Pan-American Chest Conference was being held in Lima, Peru, in the summer of 1976. Our growing family had traveled to Europe for five weeks, so South America seemed like an opportunity we shouldn't refuse. I submitted a presentation on fiberoptic bronchoscopy to justify some of the trip. When Mary and Charlie Magarrah, friends from our church, heard of our plans, they invited us over to meet a student from Colombia who was staying with them that summer. The girl's sister had spent a year with the Magarrahs, and, in turn, the Magarrahs had visited their parents in Bogota. We had a contact and put Colombia on the list of countries to visit after Peru.

Marta and Peter were twelve and ten at that time and had become seasoned travelers. They particularly enjoyed exploring archeological sites. We added Lake Titicaca; La Paz, Bolivia; Rio de Janeiro; and Manaus in the heart of the Brazilian Amazon. Because we were planning to end up in Colombia, we added a stay at a river camp near Letitia, Colombia's sliver of land that extends south to the Amazon River.

While in Lima, we had afternoons free to tour the city and some Incan and pre-Incan archeological sites. The lack of rainfall along the coast has preserved these sites in Peru better than in most places of the world.

Machu Picchu, the mountaintop fortress city near the Incan capital of Cuzco, was a special delight for our climbing youngsters. They also climbed the companion mountain, Ouija Picchu. The view of the Andes was impressive. Even more impressive was the view 1,000 feet below where the Urabamba River appeared like a ribbon in the shape of a horseshoe almost circling the smaller mountain.

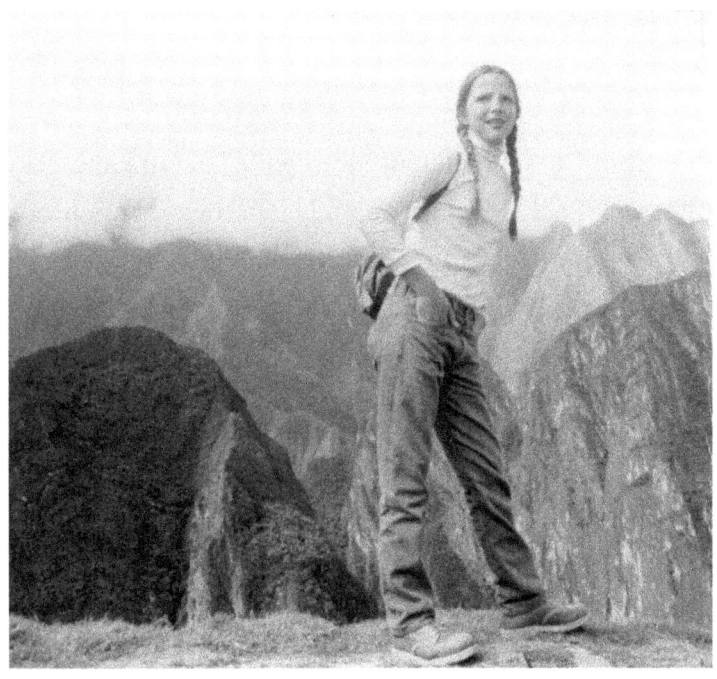

Marta at the top of Ouija Picchu overlooking the Urabamba River

ACCIDENTAL TRAFFICKING

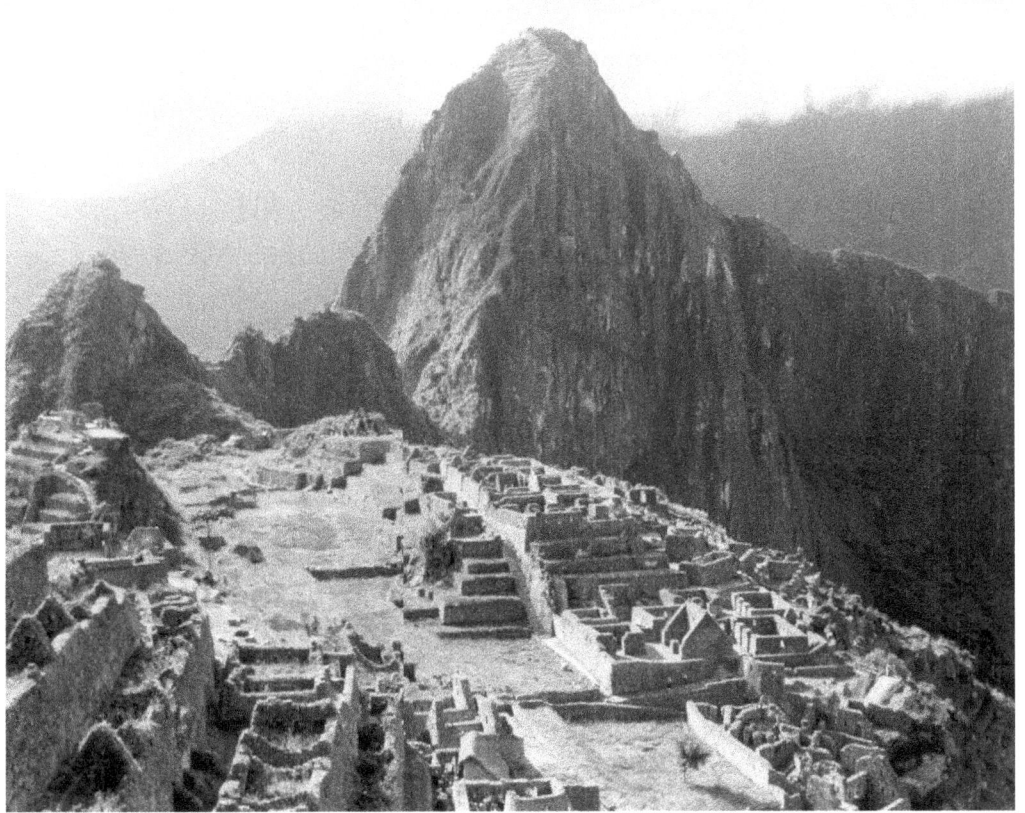

Ouija Picchu in the background of Machu Picchu

Lake Titicaca, the world's highest lake, on the border of Peru and Bolivia, with its straw boats and its short, large-lung inhabitants, taught us about adaptation at high altitudes. La Paz, Bolivia, had a dirty polluted river bisecting its center. The hotel tapwater seemed to come directly from the river. The famous Rio de Janeiro mostly lived up to its hype. Then we flew to Manaus.

Manaus is 1,000 miles from the Atlantic Ocean. Large sea-going vessels have been navigating the Amazon since the early nineteenth century. Our local guide, I will call him Raul, said he was a student and this was his part-time job. He showed us Brazil-nut trees, flooded local farmsteads, and introduced us to life on the river where we visited residents in their homes. We went pirañha fishing one morning, ate our catch for lunch, and then went swimming in the place we caught the fish.

During our stay Raul introduced us to a fifty-five-year-old Californian who was experimenting with grapefruit trees. Marta was interested in what he was doing and he insisted we visit his university laboratory. He said he was in the Peace Corps. We never were sure that he was telling the truth or whether the grapefruit research was legitimate.

Raul took us to the airport for a two-hour flight to Letitia, Colombia. The plane was small, maybe fifteen seats at most. Just before we were to board, Raul asked, "Doctor Hanson, would you mind taking a package for a friend in Letitia?" We had luggage for four, but the package was about the size of two hardcover books.

"How will I know who to give it to?"

"My friend will meet the plane. He knows your name."

What could I do but add the package to our luggage? Soon we were off flying over a jungle woven with Amazonian tributaries. Sure enough, as soon as we landed, there was a tall dark-haired male in his twenties asking, "Are you Doctor Hanson? Did Raul send a package for me?"

With this brief one-sided introduction, the package was transferred, and he disappeared into the crowd in the small river town never to be seen by us again. The drug trade between the Americas was in its infancy as far as Minnesotans were concerned. It did not occur to us until much later, after arriving home, that we had probably transported illegal drugs from Brazil to Columbia, an international border.

From Letitia we visited indigenous villages and stayed at a camp called Monkey Island. On our five-hour boat trip we saw several dugout boats carrying people and animals. One hollowed-out log boat was transporting twenty-two people!

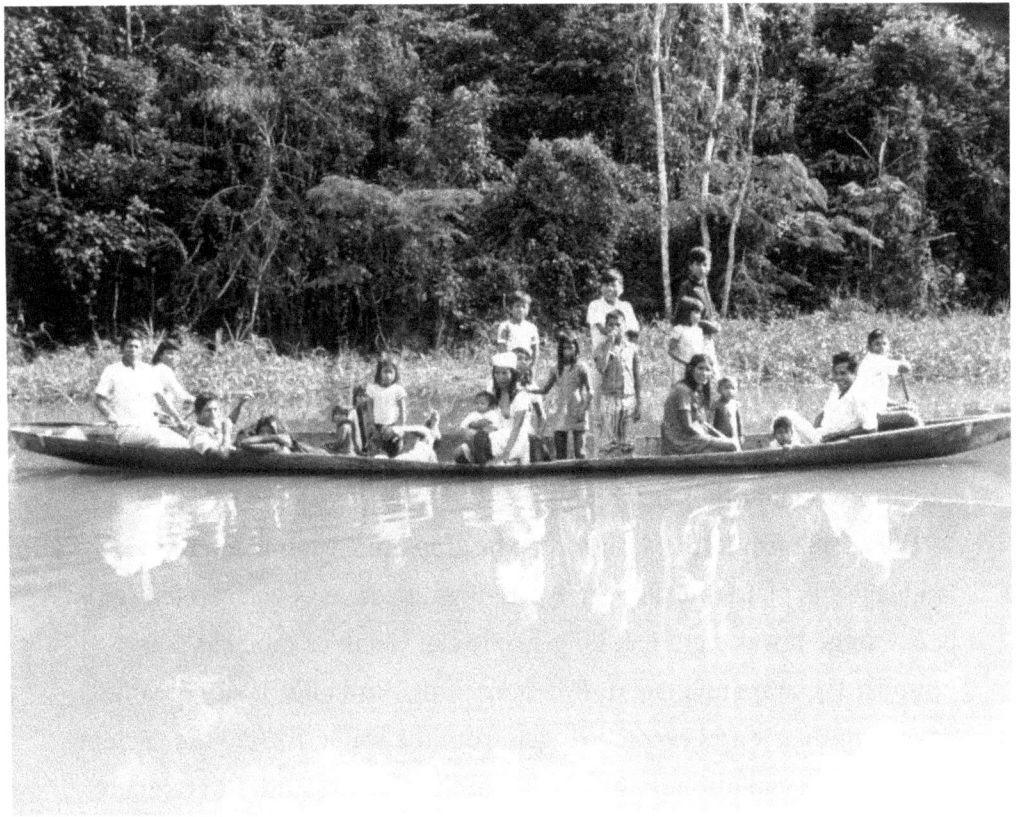

Log dugout boat with a large family

The camp consisted of several wood-framed rooms built on stilts. There were four other guests. The staff was helpful, but mostly sat around doing nothing in the heat and humidity. From the camp we made forages into the brown-water tributaries and backwaters of the Colombian Amazon. We saw monkeys, birds, huge trees, and heard animals hidden in the undergrowth.

One village had about ten dwellings, a community building, some electric lines, and a generator. The mayor told us they had problems getting their children to return to the village after they had been sent away for education. Much of rural America was experiencing the same problem at the time.

Another village was much less developed and contained only five basic shelters with open sides raised on stilts. These shelters housed up to a dozen people. We were advised to be reserved and not ask questions as these villagers were sometimes hostile to visitors. They were hunter-gatherers. A partially eaten monkey carcass lay on the floor of one dwelling — perhaps that night's meal!

The Amazon Basin is home to thousands, maybe millions, of unusual species. I was interested in a nonflying bird, the hoatzin (pronounced "watson"), one of the world's oldest living species and a link to dinosaurs. The hoatzin eats leaves and digests the cellulose, in a similar way to cows and other ruminants.

The largest fish in the Amazon is the arapaima or pirarucu in local languages. We had one alongside our dugout canoe as we traveled some backwaters. It was eight feet long. Some can weigh as much as 500 pounds. The arapaima has rudimentary lungs and gills. It can breathe oxygen in the air and extract oxygen from the water. It's like the ancient lung fish, the evolutionary link between the sea and land. Its scales are as large as silver dollars and are sold as souvenirs.

From Monkey Island and Letitia we flew to the capital, Bogota, to visit our contact from Minneapolis. The father of the Magarrahs' foreign students met us and arranged a hotel presidential suite for the price of our standard room vouchers. The next day his extended family took us to a distant park reserve for an open-fire barbecue picnic. We were near exhaustion when we found they had planned a party at their Bogota home that evening — more people, more introductions, more food, and a loud band. We discovered that we were the honored guests. The father owned a farm near Medellin, which meant nothing special to us. As we were leaving, the father asked, "Would you mind taking a small suitcase to our daughter in Minneapolis?"

"How heavy is it? What will be in it?" I asked.

"It has some clothes and books she needs."

As we left the party, he brought out a modest-sized locked suitcase that we carried back to our hotel and combined with our luggage for the trip home in the morning.

We presented our passports and clearances, but did not undergo any security checks or inspections as we checked our luggage to Minneapolis and left Bogota. A few days after arriving home we met at the Magarrahs for a meal and delivered the suitcase to the student. She thanked us and went to her room presumably to inspect her "care package" from home. We didn't see her again before we left. The next Sunday at church, Mary Magarrah said their Colombian student had unexpectedly left for New York to visit relatives. When she did not return that summer, and when she did not communicate by letter or phone, we began to put things together. We had apparently been accidental drug traffickers, not once but twice!

Before you condemn our naïveté, bear in mind this was the mid-1970s — only the beginning of what we now know to be a major illegal industry. Transit security was minimal. We presented as a trustworthy American family on vacation. No authorities asked to investigate us or our belongings.

Looking back it seems hard to believe we probably transferred illegal drugs across two international borders. We have no knowledge of what happened to the transported content or to the transporters. Raul was definitely involved. But who was the grapefruit man in Manaus? Was he involved in finding us? Was he Raul's handler? Was he connected in some way to Medellin and Bogota? Questions that can still keep us awake at night.

CHAPTER EIGHTEEN

Teaching Sex in Sunday School

What led a former schoolteacher and a young lung physician to agree to teach a sex-education class in Sunday school? In 1972 sex education in most public and private schools was Plumbing 101 with diagrams of menstruation, sperm-and-egg joining, fetal development in the uterus, and not much more. The Unitarian Universalist Association (UUA), through its Beacon Press in Boston, had developed a human-sexuality course for seventh, eighth, and ninth graders. The First Universalist Church of Minneapolis, to which we belonged, wanted to try it out. Little did we know what we were getting into.

I suppose we were viewed as an ideal couple to lead such a class. Gail had been a junior-high school teacher and had experience with the target age group. I was a practicing physician. Together, we had two preteen children, further proving we must know something about procreation and its aftereffects. Gail and I had been in the same junior-high classes on sex and the human body in our teens. We had watched films showing diagrams of sex organs with eggs releasing and sperm wiggling up channels to fight their way into an egg. Then came fertilization, uterine-egg implantation, growth of the fetus, and an eventual diagram of the delivery of a baby. I don't remember anything in that curriculum about dating relationships, emotional commitment, or values. Those topics were too controversial for schools in the early 1950s, and that was still the case when we started teaching this course in the early 1970s. I was not totally uninformed as a youth. I had spent lots of time on farms where cows, bulls, roosters, hens, and pigs mated in the barnyard and pasture.

Unitarian Universalists (UUs) in the United States at the time viewed themselves as members of a liberal religion, open to new ideas, advocates of peace, supporters of one another, and as a people committed to seeking the truth. When the headquarters in Boston put together a human-sexuality program for teens, the religion's values of open, honest, trustworthy information were presented in formats understandable and appealing. In other words, the course contained explicit visuals and discussions of human sexuality. (When we saw the materials we did have doubts.) There was no precedent to follow, but we weren't on our own. We had guideline books, some media aids in the instructors' kit, and we were hoping to develop additional parent support.

We knew that our son and daughter would be in this age group in a few years. The "birds-and-the-bees" talks were looming. Maybe leading this course would assist us in educating them when the time came. If we did it right, there might be other knowledgeable, like-minded adults around to help.

Since the program had explicit visuals that were not in common use — other than in back alleys and porn shops — we decided that each set of parents who wanted their child in the class had to attend an all-day Saturday session where we presented each unit and the accompanying materials. The exercises included "Breaking the Language Barrier." About thirty solemn adults started to list slang terms for various parts of the body associated with sex. Breasts, penis, vagina, and anus were written on flip charts. Next they went to work in small groups listing all the terms they could think of for each organ. Then someone from the small group had to read the terms to the whole group. By the end of the exercise, the parents had begun boisterously competing with one another. They were engaged and had loosened up verbally.

Other units included judging others by their appearance, listening to first sexual experiences on recordings, and close-touching experiences. Have you every tried to pass an orange from one person to another of the opposite sex without using your hands? This teenage party game using one's chin loosened the group up physically. An academic psychologist, specializing in sexuality, administered an anonymous sexual-experience survey and then presented the results. We found that within our parent group, almost all of the sexual iterations listed in the survey had been experienced by at least someone in the group. We were then ready for the visual filmstrips.

Keeping to the principles of openness, honesty, and truth, the filmstrips showed real people in bright light doing what most people do in the dark. Light- and dark-skinned couples demonstrated foreplay and intercourse between males and females and those of the same sex. The parents became very quiet.

"You're not going to show this to our kids, are you?"

"This is too much for them to absorb."

"You have to find some way to limit these visuals."

Could we present this explicit human-sexuality course that lived up to the stated values of our church to our developing kids? At the end of the day, after a lively discussion, we decided yes. But a trial class would be held Sunday afternoons. We knew that we were in competition with the public-school system and expected some local feedback, but we never expected to conflict with the federal judicial system.

The materials for this course came from the UUA and Beacon Press in Boston. We received them through the U.S. Postal Service. An aggressive U.S. district attorney in Milwaukee had convened a federal grand jury charging that pornographic materials were being sent in the U.S. mail. He requested an injunction to cease and desist and fines proposed for Beacon Press, the Unitarian Universalist Association, and anyone using the materials. What were we thinking when we agreed to lead this Sunday-school program? We didn't think that we might end up in court. We had had enough problems getting a small group of parents to agree to present this material to their kids.

While lawyers and our national organizations slogged through the court system, we plunged ahead every Sunday afternoon at 4:00 p.m. unit by unit. We used a library room that had comfortable chairs, carpeting, and muted colors. Books lined the walls, and curtains could be drawn to see the visual aids. Two boys, I'll call them Mike and Donald, were continually horsing around, laughing at some of the exercises, but actively joining in on all the activities. About halfway into the course, Donald's parents took us aside one afternoon, when they were picking him up, and told us how we had changed their weekends. They had to leave their cabin early, so he could make the class.

Our students seemed to be engaged and learning, but they were astonished to know their parents had experienced the same material. The parents, too, were becoming more comfortable and we had nearly 100 percent attendance of their sons and daughters in the class. Did this open up some communication with their parents? In some cases it did. In others, we were not so sure. Gail and I spent Saturdays reading the manuals in preparation for Sunday's class, trying to keep one step ahead of the eager teens. We finished the year feeling we had been less than perfect, but satisfied we had done our best.

The First Universalist Church in Minneapolis did not hold summer services. The Sunday-school program ended in June and began again in September. That gave the religious-education committee time to assess its offerings and plan for the coming year in September. There was consensus that the human-sexuality course should be continued.

Parents were supportive, the affected youth were ecstatic, and the courts in Milwaukee had not determined that we could not proceed. They expected that Gail and I would continue as leaders. We wanted more adults involved who could take over teaching the class when our children were the right age.

The course started the next year with four adults team-teaching, and we moved it to prime-time Sunday mornings. Parents who wanted their sons or daughters in the class were required to attend a parents' Saturday session as in the first year. The new set of parents had the same reaction as the first group. "Great course. I learned so much, but do you need to show all this to my kid?"

Our efforts did not go unnoticed in the Twin Cities. Other UU churches, societies, and fellowships followed with their own programs using the Beacon Press guidelines and tool kit. Other less liberal churches also bought the materials and went to work. We had good information that the students were talking about this course to their wider networks of friends, and a movement was forming. One Minneapolis Roman Catholic parish started a human-sexuality program for their teens based on the UU materials. Their initiative caused a division in the parish, leading some members to leave for a neighboring parish. I was never able to find out which parishes gained and which lost. Some information is best kept hidden, but I would still like to know.

Looking back, were we naïve? Yes. Were we right for the job? Yes. Did we have perfect implementation? No. Did we make a difference? Others will have to weigh in on that. Would we do it again? Of course! Gail and I benefited, our family benefited, the teens and the parents we taught thanked us for years. Did we make some inroads toward more openness when talking about human sexuality in our community? I think so. At least we made more people think about what we impart to our children and how we relate to each other. Over fifty years later, a human-sexuality class is still part of our church's Sunday-school offering.

Lastly, what happened to the attempt to limit distribution of the Beacon Press materials in federal court and to intimidate those of us trying to be more open in discussing sexuality? The charge was eventually thrown out on the basis of freedom of information protection by the U.S. Constitution. The court decided these materials were not exploiting anyone and therefore could not be deemed pornographic.

CHAPTER NINETEEN

Go by Land

In 1991 when Marta, our daughter, told us she was going from Cambridge, England, where she was studying, to Beijing, China, for a year, we were happy for her. When she wrote that she and her husband might go by land, Gail and I said, "We are going with you." We spent an exceptional month experiencing Eastern Europe, Moscow during the Gorbachev coup, a Siberian dinner with Andre, Mongolian horses and yaks, and a changed Beijing.

Marta was completing a year of graduate study at the Needham Research Institute at Cambridge University. Her mentor, Joseph Needham, a renowned scholar of Chinese science, told her the best way to understand the vast cultural difference between Europe and China was to travel there by land. Gail and I wanted to visit the Eastern European countries that were Soviet Union satellites during the Cold War, and I wanted to take a return train from Berlin to Moscow, the reverse from my Moscow to Berlin trip in 1961. The Berlin Wall had been taken down and travel by rental car and train was not difficult to arrange. The Soviet Union had weathered the unification of Germany, the liberation of Poland, a "Velvet Revolution" in Czechoslovakia, a Hungarian liberation, and Gorbachev was then in power in Moscow. Into this environment we rented a car in Berlin and started a drive through what had been East Germany. We visited Leipzig and Dresden before traveling to the Czech Republic, Prague, and then to Budapest, Hungary. We planned to drive back to Berlin, turn in the rental car, and board a Russian train to meet Marta and her husband in Moscow in five days.

After a morning run along the Danube River in Budapest, I turned on our hotel-room television to a newscast in English. Mikhail Gorbachev was under house arrest and Boris Yeltsin was standing on a tank in front of the Russian Parliament Building in Moscow. Eastern Europe was having another crisis and we were heading directly into it.

This was before smart phones and electronic note pads. The Internet was rudimentary and was used primarily by university researchers and the military. The only access to urgent personal communications was through landline telephones or telegraphs. When we finally talked to Marta, we decided to talk again in two days, when Gail and I were scheduled to be in Berlin and Marta in Stockholm.

The Hungarians were reluctant to sell us gas for our trip north through the Carpathian mountains and into Poland. The Poles were more withdrawn. The Soviet Union was their main supplier of fuel and the political uncertainty in Moscow gave them great reluctance to sell foreigners any gasoline. Their palpable anxiety fueled our anxiety and we could get no car-radio news in English. Two days after hearing the broadcast in Budapest, as we drove into Berlin, we found a BBC station. The first words we heard were, "Isn't it nice that we can now talk about something other than the events in Moscow." What? We wanted news of Moscow and the station was pivoting to other world news.

We settled for a night in Berlin, talked to Marta, who was now in Stockholm, and decided to keep to our plan to meet in Moscow. The next morning Gail and I filled a new duffel bag with dried and canned foods that would be needed for a two-week journey across Russia, Siberia, Mongolia, and northern China. That afternoon we boarded a Russian train for my 28-hour "return trip" to Moscow.

The train had no food, and we started to dig into our pack. In Moscow our sense of anxiety increased. The restaurants had big menus, but only one or two choices were available. We couldn't exchange money, and we were scheduled to be traveling for a week by train across Siberia.

Moscow had changed since I had visited in 1961. Lenin and Stalin were no longer displayed in a mausoleum along the Kremlin's outside wall. The Russian flag had replaced the Soviet flag flying over the Kremlin's central building. Basil's Cathedral on Red Square had been repaired and open to the public. But the GUM department store had kept its place across Red Square opposite the Kremlin. We could walk around inside the Kremlin walls and visit the domed Orthodox churches that contained the tombs of past czars. The subway was operating, but there were few cars.

We went to where the tanks-against-rows-of-civilians conflict had taken place five days earlier. Rotating resisters had lined up five deep in front of the Russian Parliament that they call the "White House." We met a family who had participated in the citizen confrontation. The Soviet tanks they faced were gone, but makeshift barricades of furniture, mattresses, sticks, and any other junk available remained. The barricades reminded me of the depiction of barricades during the French Revolution in the musical *Les Miserables*. A main thoroughfare near the White House was still closed to traffic. A makeshift memorial to the three resisters killed in the conflict was piled with fading flowers and attracted other walkers. A transition of geopolitical power had taken place. The Communist world was being transformed.

DO NO HARM

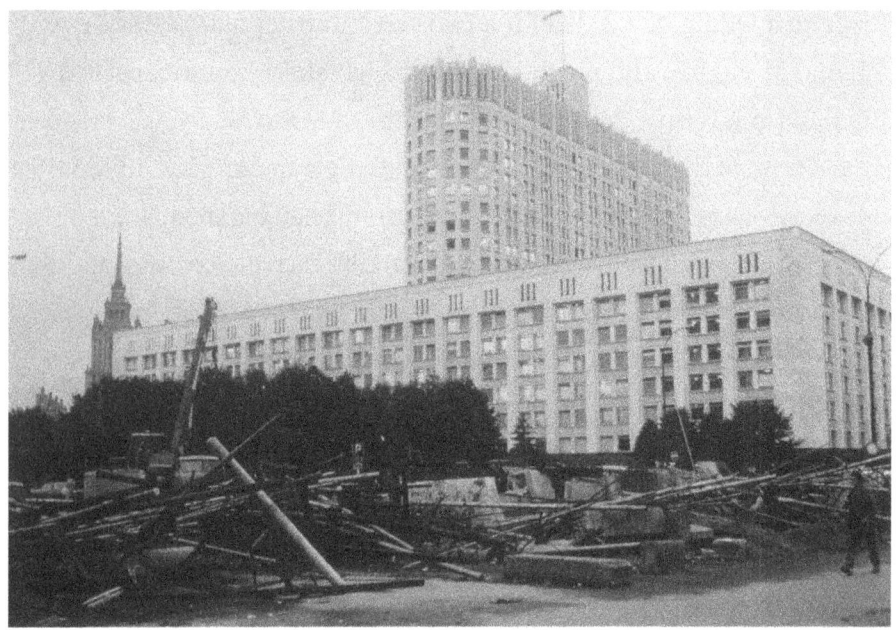

Russian White House in Moscow with barricades in front

We boarded the train for Novosibirsk for a two-day ride across the Russian countryside. The first thing we saw in Novosibirsk was a large building being built with workers who were supervised by armed guards. Prison labor was building a new hotel near the train station.

We were told our hotel was two years old. There were some rough edges, but it served us well after two nights on the trans-Siberian train. Novosibirsk was a sister-city to Minneapolis, and we had a school teacher to contact. She had us speak English to classrooms in her school and took us near a scientific research center that foreigners were not allowed to visit. Then she took us to what she called a supermarket that served the research center's population. Almost all the shelves were empty, except for one small area occupied by some poorly wrapped candy. A few Russians walked into the store, saw there were no other goods for sale that day, and walked out.

We invited our guide to have dinner with us, but she never arrived. She may have feared the possibilities of a dinner in the new hotel.

The hotel dining room was on the top floor. When the four of us arrived, several tables were filled and a band was playing Western-style music. A large table of birthday celebrants was positioned between us and the band at the front of the room. Russian champagne was inexpensive, and the hotel provided a full menu. This was a great contrast to Moscow and the train. Gail and I were tired of eating nonperishable foods from our duffel bag. We ordered our meals and noticed the birthday table had many candles. We purchased two to enlighten our first good meal since leaving Berlin and Stockholm.

Then, a man at a two-person table on my left hit the woman he was with across the face and knocked her to the floor. She was bruised but got up, as the manager came to settle things down. Their conversation in Russian ended, the couple sat down at their table, and they began to eat as the band finished their song and took a break.

We settled back to our meal discussing what had just happened. Then we heard some musical strains that sounded like a beginner practicing on a new instrument. When I looked up, there were two people from the birthday table playing on the bands' instruments. Now, the band hurriedly returned and chased the party-goers off the bandstand and back to their table.

As we started to settle back to our meal, I heard a crash. There followed a second crash before I realized the party-table members were sailing small plates toward the band. The manager came and required everyone at the birthday table to leave. As the band continued playing, the birthday party began leaving. The honored guest picked up her large bouquet of white roses and several of the still-burning candles they had purchased. As she walked out of the room, her hair caught on fire, singeing the side of her face.

The fire was quickly extinguished and most of the party left the room. Then a young man from the party came over and sat down at our table. He introduced himself in English as Andre, and apologized for the disturbance. He explained that they were having a birthday party for his fiancée. We had never experienced a dinner quite like it. For years since we have called this "Our Dinner with Andre."

We traveled two days and nights from Novosibirsk by train to the city of Irkutsk, which is located near Lake Baikal, the largest freshwater lake in the world (by volume of water: Lake Superior has a larger surface area). After our dinner with Andre, everything else was anticlimactic.

To get to Mongolia we changed trains in Ulan-Ude on the southeast side of Lake Baikal. The new train ran once a week through Mongolia to Beijing. In Ulan Bator we visited a friend who was serving in the Peace Corps. Mongolia was extracting itself from the Soviet influence, and the people were uncertain of their future. It was another country on edge.

We spent a day in a small yurt village that housed an extended family. I went out back to inspect their corral, which contained about thirty horses. One of the younger men was milking one of the mares. Inside the central yurt we were served local delicacies followed by fermented mare's-milk called koumiss. It tasted like clotted Bulgarian buttermilk mixed with yogurt. Outside two girls demonstrated their horse skills, and we all rode a yak.

We enjoyed our Mongolian stay, but didn't have time to wait a week for the next train to Beijing. We were scheduled to fly on what might have been the only jet in Mongolia. At least we saw no other jets or large planes when we arrived at the airport. We taxied up the mountainside runway, turned around, and started downhill on a pitted bumpy piece of concrete that shook the plane to its core before it was airborne. Our course took us directly over the Great Wall of China. It was built to keep the Mongolians out of China, but it offered no resistance to our plane or to the Mongolians for that matter! From the air we could see several other crumbling walls that carry their own histories.

GO BY LAND

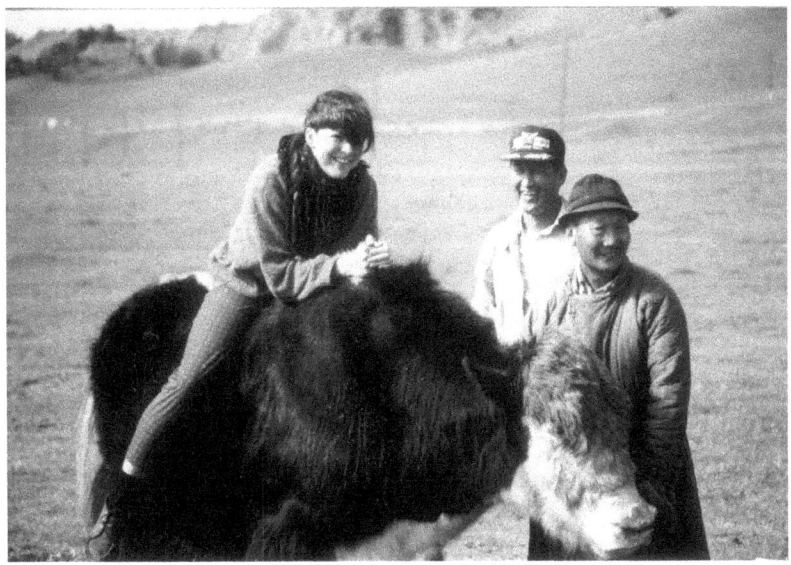

Marta, our Chinese scholar, on a Mongolian yak

Beijing had undergone a cultural shift since we had been there in 1981. Masses of bicycles with silent riders in grey, blue, or green Maoist-era jackets had been replaced by noisy, fume-producing cars crowding the pedestrians who walked the street edges. Drab, colorless clothing had been replaced by miniskirted women in colorful dresses and high-heeled shoes hurrying from shop to shop searching for the perfect fruit or vegetable. Street venders cooked food at the edge of the crowded streets. The floor mat in our high-rise hotel elevator said Tuesday. The next day it said Wednesday.

In the weeks we had been traveling from Berlin to Beijing, a seismic geopolitical shift had started to take place with minimal loss of life. The independence movement in Eastern Europe was extending to Russia, Soviet Asia, and Mongolia. We had visited several of the long-forbidden Soviet satellite countries, glimpsed a major transition in Moscow, experienced the vastness of Siberia and Mongolia, and witnessed an evolution toward capitalism in Beijing. Going by land had made all the difference in our understanding of the cultural and geopolitical differences between Europe and China.

A Physician's Life

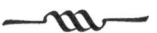

CHAPTER TWENTY

Pulmonary Medicine

While in medical school I had to consider what I wanted to do with a medical degree. Did I want to be a pediatrician like my uncle Carl? Did I want to be a general practitioner and start practicing medicine after a year of internship and obtaining a license? Or did I want to take advanced training to be a medical specialist? These are decisions all medical students need to make.

I was most interested in the broad fields of medicine as I started clinical rotations at the University of Minnesota in 1961. I had tested an interest in research at Dartmouth and found that I wanted more human interaction. I liked teaching, but physicians in academic settings who were primarily teachers had difficulty advancing their careers. During the two clinical years of medical school, I found internal medicine most suited to my interests and personal preferences. I could sense that general practice was undergoing change. No residency training for family practice had been established in the Midwest. Also, I did not like working with dying children and their parents at the university.

I had been invited to a surgically oriented student group who met in the surgical-faculty homes. I became the president of the group as a senior, but one of the senior surgical professors said, "Hanson, with your ideas about medical care, you sound like someone suited for public health." My interests in the health of populations did not fit well with a surgical career. (I later met this same professor in court, which I describe in another chapter.)

Internal medicine in the early 1960s was a broad specialty caring for adults. At teaching centers some individual internists narrowed their interests to one organ like the heart or one disease such as tuberculosis, but there were no defined and accredited subspecialty disciplines. Formal internal-medicine subspecialties with national boards didn't develop until the 1970s. This was the medical environment I was entering in 1961–1963 when I needed to decide on my career course.

I felt internal medicine fit my needs and interests, but I wanted to be well grounded in general medicine. I chose to take a rotating internship that I described in a previous chapter, "The General." I wanted a "liberal arts" education in general medicine before specializing.

As I was completing my internal-medicine training at the University of Minnesota and the Minneapolis VA Hospital, I began looking for positions in the community. I had decided not to pursue an academic-research-and-teaching career. My heart was in delivering care, and private multispecialty-group practice was my preference. I had been exposed to group practice at Dartmouth and at the Minneapolis VA Hospital. I thought I could be comfortable working and continuing to learn from being in a group of physicians with different specialties.

Physicians who had served in WWI formed a multispecialty group in Minneapolis in 1921 called the Nicollet Clinic. A similarly minded group of WWII veterans in 1951 formed a multispecialty group in a western Minneapolis suburb that they called the St. Louis Park Medical Center. Both groups had been successful, and in 1971, after I interviewed, I decided to join the St. Louis Park group. They said they needed another pulmonologist, and I decided to train for the position. This was before there were formal fellowships in pulmonary disease in the Twin Cities. Gail and I were not interested in relocating to another city with our family, so I took a junior-staff position at the VA Hospital in the pulmonary department and began focusing on becoming a pulmonary-medicine specialist. When I went back to talk to the leaders of the St. Louis Park Medical Center a year later, they said they had already hired another pulmonologist. They were willing to add me to the department on the expectation that I would also practice general internal medicine. I didn't have much salary leverage when I received a contract.

I had previous experience with using fiberoptic scopes to investigate the gastrointestinal tract while at the VA Hospital. Japanese physicians had adapted fiberoptics to scopes that could be passed into the lungs. No one in the Twin Cities was using the new bronchoscopes at the time. I was interested in expanding my diagnostic capacity and urged the pulmonary department at the VA to order one of the new instruments. It arrived two weeks before I was due to join the St. Louis Park Medical Center in July of 1971. There were no practice models or instructional courses to take, so I tried it out in the morgue. Thus began my learning in the subspecialization of pulmonary medicine.

My new organization was willing to purchase one of the new fiber-optic bronchoscopes if the surgeons, who did bronchoscopies using a rigid instrument in an operating room, supported the idea. I would be competing for patients with the chest and the ear-nose-and-throat surgeons. The scope was approved with the expectation I would report my experience to the group in a year.

The new instrument was a vast improvement. A patient's airway could be visualized better and biopsies and brushing specimens could be taken under direct vision. When I presented my report to my colleagues, I also had photographs of bronchial cancers to go along with chest X-rays and pathological tissue specimens. No one else in the Twin Cities was using this revolutionary equipment. After I presented my experience to the Minneapolis Society of Internal Medicine, I began receiving consults from physicians outside our group. One of those cases is discussed in the next chapter.

Fiberoptic bronchoscopy was not the only innovation that impacted pulmonary medicine after I finished my formal training. I had learned to biopsy the inside lining of the chest, the pleura, while at the VA. In a rare case, I had also tried to biopsy large lung masses with large liver-biopsy needles. Pulmonary physicians wanted to get tissue from patients with diffuse lung disease and small lung nodules, but the risk of doing so with large needles usually outweighed the benefits. I went to a meeting in London where a Brompton Hospital physician, Dr. Steel, was using a drill-like needle that he had reported in the medical literature. The demonstration procedure caused the patient's lung to collapse, and I never used the "Steel" needle. Its use faded as more of us became comfortable using bronchial forceps with fluoroscopy for diffuse lung disease and thinner needles for lung masses and nodules.

These innovations in pulmonary medicine changed the diagnostic practices in chest medicine tremendously. With the fine-needle and the new bronchoscopic techniques, often using real-time radiographic or ultrasound localization, exploratory chest surgery for an unknown diagnosis became rare.

I learned two other interventional procedures to aid in the therapy of lung diseases. Large airway obstruction, usually from cancers in inoperable patients, was occasionally a difficult problem. I went to San Diego for a practical course in using lasers to remove the obstructing tissue. We started using the technique at Methodist Hospital in 1984. Two years later I took a course in pleuroscopy in Indianapolis. Inoperable malignancies of the lung or pleural space surrounding the lung can cause fluid buildup compressing the functioning lung. Direct vision of the pleura with a scope could result in better outcomes than some of the indirect treatment methods we were using. When I requested operating privileges at the hospital, I received approval with the stipulation that a chest surgeon be immediately available. About that time our cardiothoracic surgeons became more interested in and willing to perform these procedures on these complicated cases, and I was relieved.

Besides these interventional procedures, there were many other changes that challenged and improved the capacity of pulmonologists. Blood-gas measurements were a research tool at the VA hospital as I started training in pulmonary medicine in 1969. Pulmonary function tests were not easily obtained, there was no intensive care unit, and ventilators were unreliable. Critical care units, specialized nurses, dependable ventilators, and respiratory therapists have made major improvements in what we have to offer patients. The advances in managing severely ill and injured patients has led to the development of a new specialty, critical care, with all the discipline and credentialing of a new medical specialty.

A similar evolution has taken place in sleep medicine. I first heard of the "snort syndrome" as I was completing my training in 1971. There was no formal discipline encompassing sleep disorders. The symptoms of sleep apnea were later tied to central airway obstruction during sleep due to oral-muscle relaxation, often complicated by obesity. Airway access was the expertise of pulmonologists and another new specialty developed around sleep disorders and their treatments.

These are some of the advances I have experienced since I completed training in pulmonary medicine. Interventional diagnostic equipment has revolutionized pulmonary diagnosis. Intensive care capacities have saved many lives and changed how and when some people die. Critical care medicine has challenged how we deliver and how we pay for health care and has raised ethical issues we didn't have when I started. And then there is sleep medicine, a discipline I couldn't have imagined in 1971.

I have been honored to practice with a group of highly motivated physicians and am grateful for the colleagues who allowed me to join their multispecialty-group practice. Their motto was to hire the best doctors they could attract, and I continue to have great respect for the physicians with whom I have had the privilege to work. I always felt that when l was off-call or out of town, my patients would be treated as well or better than when I was available. That has been a great comfort and allowed a life-balance for which I am sincerely grateful.

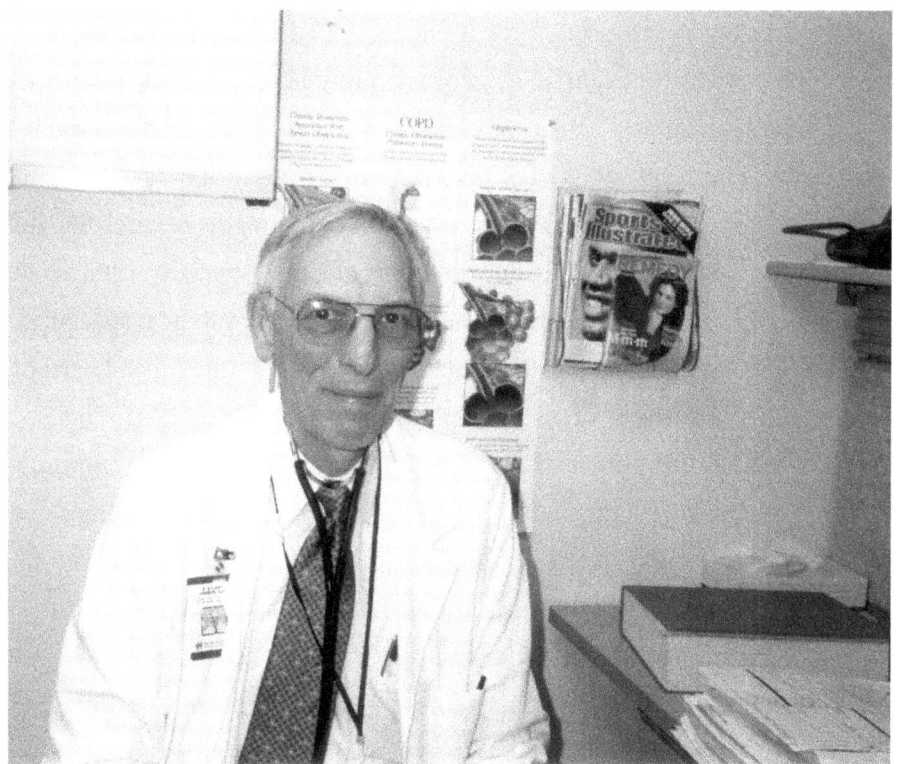

Exam room photo taken by a patient, 2002

CHAPTER TWENTY-ONE

My Practice Meets the Law

It was a day like many other days practicing at my medical office in St. Louis Park, Minnesota, a first-ring suburb of Minneapolis. I had made hospital rounds and seen my morning-office patients when a receptionist said there was a man in the waiting room who insisted on seeing me. This was in 1974, long before Minnesota medical facilities were concerned about personal safety in our buildings. When I met the man in our waiting room, he said, "Are you Dr. Arthur Stuart Hanson?"

"Yes, I am."

"I represent the Hennepin County District Court and am here to serve you this summons. Please sign here that you received it."

Thus began my first encounter with the law as a defendant.

The 1970s were a litigious era for those practicing medicine. Physician organizations like the American Medical Association were pushing for limits on liability and court procedures to reduce frivolous suits. Professional-liability insurance was a significant cost for a medical practice. Now I was being pulled into this environment.

It took me the rest of the day to absorb what had happened. I had a full schedule of patients to see before I had the time to read the packet of difficult-to-interpret documents. By evening I had determined that myself, three other physicians, and Group Health of Minnesota, a cooperative-insurance plan and healthcare delivery organization, were being sued by the family of a deceased patient we had cared for two years previously. For me — a young physician three years into private practice — the lawsuit was devastating.

I remembered the case well. She was a 27-year-old, nonsmoking, married woman who presented to a Group Health Plan outpatient office with respiratory symptoms. Before I saw her, a general internist had initially treated her symptomatically. When she did not improve, an X-ray was taken. It showed what appeared to be pneumonia in the upper lobe of the right lung. Antibiotics led to some symptom improvement, but the lung appeared worse on another X-ray. An independent chest surgeon was consulted and he performed a rigid bronchoscopy. (At the time, the standard of care was to inspect the trachea and central bronchial tubes with a rigid, hollow, silver-like tube passed though the vocal cords in an operating room under general anesthesia.)

The chest surgeon found no abnormalities, but he could not see the bronchus going to the right upper lobe due to the nearly 180-degree angle the bronchus takes in relation to the trachea and right main-stem bronchus. Based on the X-ray, he knew this was where the problem was, but he could not get to it with the rigid instrument.

I went through a standard pulmonary evaluation and reviewed her X-rays. This was long before computer-assisted imaging such as CT, MRI, or ultrasound scans were available. I saw no mass to suggest cancer. The lung process had presented as an upper-lobe pneumonia, but now the whole upper lobe was collapsed. A skin test for tuberculosis was applied, and outpatient fiberoptic bronchoscopy was scheduled for the next day, with the referring surgeon assisting.

MY PRACTICE MEETS THE LAW

With the flexible instrument, we found that the trachea and other central airways were normal except for the right upper lobe. We found that the bronchus was narrowed, thickened, and inflamed, but there was no tumor mass or foreign body. Biopsies, brushings, photos, and cultures for bacteria, fungus, and tuberculosis were taken. We hoped to make a specific diagnosis in the next few days. When we received the first reports, no objective diagnosis could be made. Could this be a fungus or tuberculosis? Those cultures would take weeks to grow.

I went to see the patient at the hospital across town where she was hospitalized to read her TB-skin test. To my surprise it was positive. On further reflection the patient remembered she had worked with two TB patients the previous year. We still had no diagnosis, but we had some leads.

I recommended starting treatment for tuberculosis while we waited weeks for the TB cultures to grow. If no infectious diagnosis could be made and the X-ray shadows had not improved, then I would recommend a surgical exploration. The treating doctors followed my recommendations.

I didn't hear anything more for about a month, when I learned she had gone to the University of Minnesota where another rigid bronchoscopy had found invasive cancer in a random biopsy of normal-appearing tracheal tissue. She and her husband decided to get treatment at the university. I had heard nothing further about her until the day I was summoned to court.

I was shaken; my confidence was challenged. I had done my best, and now I had cause to doubt my decisions. In the next days and weeks, I poured over my records. Should I have done things differently? Did any delay in diagnosis make a difference in the final fatal outcome? I talked to the referring surgeon. I received a call from a lawyer hired by our liability-insurance companies to represent us. I wrote a case summary. My nights were fitful. I thought about the case anytime I was alone.

Eventually, I was asked to give a deposition. I presented my side of the case. A court recorder took down everything I said. My lawyer and several other lawyers were present. I gave my credentials, my summary of the case, and my thinking. Then the plaintiff's lawyer cross-examined me.

"You are a pulmonologist, is that right?"

"Yes."

"Who are the leading authorities in your field?"

"There are 10,000 pulmonologists in the United States. Each one has specialized medical training and experience."

"Do you recognize one or two who stand out above the others?"

"There are many highly specialized physicians."

"Have you written any papers?"

"Yes, I submitted a bibliography."

"In this case you thought she had tuberculosis?"

"No, that was one of the possibilities."

And so it went for almost two hours. Everything I said was now part of the court record, a part of the fact-finding process that would grind on for the next eighteen months. About a week later I read my deposition. It read terribly. It recorded the way I talked, with all my "uhs" and "ahs." My lawyer thought it was fine. He assured me there was nothing damaging in the deposition, and that I should not lose any more sleep.

I read the other physicians' depositions. The radiologist's seemed straightforward but also read poorly. The surgeon's read like the others, but revealed the thoughtful, confident, self-assured surgeon that I knew him to be. The primary physician's deposition more or less put the case in the surgeon's and my court. When the patient didn't get better after his initial treatment, he had referred her to specialists and followed their advice. So far it looked as though the surgeon and I were the responsible parties.

Any plaintiff bringing a professional-liability action needs expert witnesses. We waited to see who that would be. Who would say we had not followed sound medical procedures? Who would say we did not meet the community standard of care?

Months went by as we waited for the fact-finding process to end. Then one day I received a packet in the mail from the lawyer the insurance company had assigned to the primary-care specialist, the surgeon, and me. It contained a letter asking for a phone call after I had read the opinion letter (called an interrogatory) from the plaintiff's expert witness.

The interrogatory letter was from an internationally recognized cardio-thoracic surgeon from the University of Minnesota. He was a surgery professor I'd had in medical school. As students, we feared him. He was an imposing figure with large hands, dark hair, a stern face, and a stout body on a six-foot frame. His weekly surgical conference was something to be endured. He would pick apart a case presentation no matter how hard the student had studied and prepared. Fear, intimidation, and harassment were his methods of teaching. He was said to do the same in the operating room. Now he was a professional witness against us.

I called our lawyer and said, "We have a bully here."

"What do you mean?"

"He is a formidable physician and a good surgeon, but we can't let him get away with an opinion that doesn't fit the facts. I don't understand why he is doing this. We have to defend this case."

"Are you willing to go to court and stand up to this expert? You and the referring chest surgeon will be the key defense witnesses."

"Right now I say yes, but I want to talk to the surgeon."

When I did, he had a similar reaction. The reasoning of the plaintiff's witness — that any treating physician would know from the beginning that this was not pneumonia but a condition that required early surgical intervention — was divergent from what we did, and our opinion had not changed. We resolved not to offer any settlement. If they wanted to go to court, we were ready.

More months went by, but finally, a court date was set. I began another comprehensive review of all the medical data, the depositions, the opposing expert's opinion letter, and several defense-lawyer conversations. We had three defense lawyers involved: one representing the radiologist and two representing the primary-care physician, the chest surgeon, me, and Group Health Plan. Several days before the court date, we were notified that the plaintiff's lawyer planned to put the four defending physicians on the witness stand. Were we ready?

"Everyone, please rise."

The black-robed judge entered through a door in the back of the wood-paneled courtroom. I thought, "He has come from his office, and we were now in his examining room."

He took his seat behind an impressive desk on a raised platform that obstructed any view of what he had in front of him. Even seated he was five feet above us. We sat behind a wooden rail with our table and chairs facing his bench. A slightly raised witness stand was to our right. Farther to the right were two rows of chairs in an empty jury box. The formalities had begun.

"Please be seated," said the judge. "We are here today to hear a complaint about the way a patient was treated by doctors working for Group Health of Minnesota. The whole story will be forthcoming as the case is presented. We will now begin jury selection."

For the rest of the morning potential jurors filed into the room and were questioned by both sets of lawyers and the judge. There were questions about their education and their work backgrounds. Did they know the plaintiffs? The defendants? Had they heard about the case? Would they listen carefully to the testimony? Could they give an objective judgment? The lawyers on both sides then removed the jurors they didn't want. During a recess, our defense team discussed those who remained. This was all new to me and was more formal and detailed than any workers' compensation hearing I had attended or any TV show I had seen. Finally, six jury members and one alternate were selected and empaneled.

Our lawyers moved to remove the three treating physicians from the case. "Counselors, approach the bench," said the judge, which led to a conference out of my earshot.

"Not granted," he replied.

Next the radiologist's lawyer moved to have his client removed from the case. I thought this was odd since we had just lost our motion. There was another call to approach the bench. Another conference, then another ruling.

"Granted."

I was stunned. What was going on? (Later, I found out that the plaintiff had no expert witness to counter the decisions made by the radiologist. Therefore, he could go back to reading X-rays and sleeping well at night. Now there were three of us defending our practice.)

The opening statements delivered from each side seemed to drone on. They were the same words I had heard and read so many times over the past two years. My mind was going numb. Then the plaintiff's lawyer called the first witness.

The primary-care physician had trained at the Mayo Clinic as a general internist before being employed at Group Health. He had dark hair, greying sideburns, and a hint of an afternoon shadow on his face. His round face and forehead perspiration made him appear nervous. He had trouble focusing on the plaintiff's attorney's questions, and his answers were indecisive and muddled. By the time our attorney had a chance to help him during cross-examination, it was too late.

We were not off to a good start. At the recess, our lawyers asked what we wanted to do. The plaintiffs were offering to settle. I looked at the chest surgeon, whom we expected would be called next. He asked me what I thought. The trial had just begun, and I was not ready to give in. We resolved to forge ahead.

On the witness stand, after establishing his credentials and his involvement with the patient, the chest surgeon was asked why he did not operate when he couldn't make a diagnosis with the rigid bronchoscope.

"I did not want to operate on this young woman unless it was necessary," he replied. "I had read articles about a new flexible bronchoscope that might help me make a diagnosis before subjecting her to surgery. I was ready to send this young, nonsmoking woman anywhere in the country, if it would help her. I wanted the best possible care and the best possible consultant available. A physician at the University of Iowa was using the new instrument, but none of my colleagues had any experience with his team. Then I learned Dr. Stuart Hanson had over a year's experience and had reported his work to the Minneapolis Society of Internal Medicine. I chose the best consultant I knew and that was Dr. Hanson."

What was happening? I was being set up by my own colleague!

There was a pause. The plaintiff's lawyers asked for a ten-minute recess. Our team retreated to a side conference room behind the jury box. I told our surgeon that I felt uncomfortable with the accolades he had used to describe me. He said that was the way he felt. Our lawyers were reassuring and said I would likely be next. We all were anxious when we returned to the courtroom.

"Everyone please be seated," the judge said. "Please proceed with your case, Counsel."

"The plaintiff calls . . ." He named the cardio-thoracic surgeon from the University of Minnesota; my former professor; the writer of the interrogatory letter.

What? Not me? What was going on?

"You are the expert witness in this case. Will you give us your background and your experience treating lung diseases."

We knew he would eventually be on the stand, and we had a plan. The chest surgeon and I were more convinced than ever that we had done nothing wrong. The patient had a bad disease and an unfortunate outcome, but we would not have altered our recommendations.

We moved our chairs up to the rail, as close to the witness stand as we could get. From there we fixed our gazes on the speaker. In a sense we were challenging him in a court of law in the same way he had challenged us with his opinion letter.

"Would you read your interrogatory response?" After the letter was read the plaintiff's attorney asked, "Is it still your expert opinion that the Group Health doctors and their consultants did not meet the standard of this community in caring for this patient?"

There was a pause. We kept our eyes fixed on the witness. He made eye contact. The pause continued. Now the courtroom was silent, and everyone's attention was drawn to his answer.

"Would you please repeat the question?" he asked.

The court recorder read the question again. "Is it still your expert opinion that the Group Health doctors and their consultants did not meet the standard of this community in caring for this patient?"

"I cannot say that."

The judge interrupted. "You realize your expert opinion is the center of this case. Your letter states the doctors did not meet the standards of this community. Is that your opinion now?"

Another pause. Finally he responded,

"It is no longer my opinion."

The judge asked, "Will the counselors approach the bench?"

After a long private conference with the lawyers from both sides, he said, "Jurors, you are excused. I will meet you in the jury room in a few minutes to explain what has happened."

Then he explained to the rest of the courtroom: "The court rules in favor of the defense. The plaintiff has failed to show cause. This matter is closed. Court dismissed."

We had defended ourselves without presenting a defense. I was elated, but shaken. I'd had my day in court without saying a word. The law had taken two years to grind through its processes to an abrupt conclusion.

I went over to greet the patient's husband, whom I knew from the day I did the bronchoscopy on his wife. He told me she had wanted him and her family to know: Would the outcome have been different if her illness had been treated another way? He said now he had closure, and he thanked us for caring for his wife.

The plaintiff's expert witness came over. "I really wasn't out to get you, doctors," he said. "I wanted to get that socialist Group Health outfit. But I couldn't do it in court." I wasn't going to ask for further explanation, but he was known to be against doctors who shared patients in multispecialty-group practices. He also had spoken out against a cooperative community-owner practice that he considered socialism.

The bully had spoken! That was the last time I talked to him. Twenty years later, after he retired, a cardio-thoracic surgeon on our medical staff asked if we could hire this physician as a part-time, surgical professor. I was then the president of the research and education arm of Park Nicollet Health Services, the merged successor to the multispecialty group I joined in 1971. I thought we could arrange for credentials in our hospital, but he wanted to be paid for his services. I was never able to obtain the funds.

My initial experience with medicine and the law was an emotional trial. The years of uncertainty, the repeated reviews of the case, the interaction with lawyers, and the experience in a courtroom was a life-changing experience.

I had grown as a physician. My confidence in making decisions became stronger. I gained a better understanding of the role that honest, complex information could play in disputes. My respect for the law and its professionals grew each time I had legal encounters. I had two more summons in the next ten years. During the fact-finding process, both cases were dropped. These and other physicians' cases that were honestly and vigorously defended led to a reduction in frivolous medical-liability suits in Minnesota. From my experiences,

I developed confidence that, slow as the process might be, the courts could get it right.

As the years passed, I was asked to review other legal cases and I testified as an expert witness. I tried to do my best. I insisted on reading all the medical data, doctors' notes, nurses' notes, imaging files, pathological specimens, and any other data about the case. I was an expert witness for plaintiffs, defendants, and corporations. I always gave my best opinion, sometimes telling lawyers they were unlikely to defend their case successfully and should settle. But also I was willing to go to court to testify against cases that represented bad practice, or when I felt compelled to defend practice that was appropriate. It was hard work, and I did not seek it. But when it came, I could not refuse. The judicial system treated me well, and I still believe in the rule of law and that the courts will be fair and just as they sort through evidence and make their judgments.

(First published in *Minnesota Medicine* as "Medical Practice Meets the Law: A physician recalls his first brush with the legal system," November/December 2017, p. 20–25. Reprinted by permission.)

CHAPTER TWENTY-TWO

Stillwater Prison

When Frank MacDonald, the Chief of Pulmonary Medicine at the Minneapolis VA Hospital, asked me to join him on a consultation at the Minnesota State Prison in Stillwater, Minnesota, I had no idea what was to come. A prisoner had been diagnosed with tuberculosis, and the prison officials needed medical expertise. I was a fellow in pulmonary-medicine training, and Dr. MacDonald was my professor and mentor. He thought it might be a good experience for me to join him.

The initial visit to the prison was interesting. The guards at the front gate knew we were coming and let us through. We passed through two more barred gates, which closed behind us. I had never been in a prison and assumed we would be let out whenever we wanted. Most of the men we met did not have that opportunity.

We met with the general practitioner who had requested the consultation. He led us through the main cell blocks to another set of gates to meet the warden, Jack Young. Warden Young was a statewide personality. He had been interviewed frequently on newscasts, especially when inmates made escape attempts. In the previous two years, several escapes had occurred from St. Paul where sick inmates were hospitalized. The issue was a source of political concern for the state.

I recognized the warden immediately. I estimated him to be in his early fifties. His light brown hair and pleasant, welcoming smile made me feel more comfortable in the prison. He thanked us for coming, discussed the prison's problem, and asked for a timely report.

Dr. MacDonald and I met the medically isolated patient. He was not severely ill, but we recommended treatment in a prison hospital where he could be safely isolated and his therapy closely observed. We also recommended skin tests for all inmates and follow-up on any positives. I was designated to do the follow-up the next week.

A few days later I had a call from the prison doctor. "We've got a problem. Five inmates have positive skin tests."

"Get chest X-rays, routine blood counts, and serum-transaminase tests on each man, and I will see them on Thursday afternoon." Thus, I then began making weekly visits to the prison for the next five years.

None of the skin-test-positive inmates had any respiratory symptoms, and their chest X-rays were negative. All five were started on standard prophylactic TB therapy, which at the time was nine months of a single TB drug called Isoniazid (abbreviated to INH). The concept was to prevent active contagious tuberculosis by giving Isoniazid treatment prophylactically.

I had been concerned with the side effect of INH on the liver. Most TB specialists felt it was more important to prevent clinical tuberculosis with INH therapy than to worry about a drug-induced mild liver reaction. But there had been some deaths associated with INH therapy, so I did a blood test, called liver transaminase, after a month of therapy. Three of the patients had elevated transaminase levels in their blood. Now what to do?

For patients at the VA Hospital with suggestive evidence of hepatitis, I had performed liver biopsies that showed significant changes. The question became how to treat individuals who are incarcerated. Could they give informed consent to an invasive procedure?

With the written consent of the affected inmates and the support of the warden, I performed liver biopsies on the three inmates who now became my patients. All showed signs of hepatitis. The Isoniazid treatment was stopped in two of the cases, and all three were followed closely with chest X-rays and blood tests for the next year. All of the hepatitis patients returned to normal after INH was stopped, and none of the five inmates with positive TB-skin tests developed active tuberculosis.

One day as I was finishing my afternoon seeing patients, the prison physician asked, "Would you consider becoming the prison internist? I am having trouble managing several inmates with diabetes and inmates complaining of chest pain."

Inmates had been faking heart attacks, which led to emergency-ambulance runs from the prison to St. Paul, twenty-five miles away. After they were admitted two guards were required at the bedside twenty-four hours a day. Some inmates would attempt escapes. It seemed every few months another escape attempt, successful or unsuccessful, was in the Minneapolis and the St. Paul news.

Also diabetic inmates were manipulating their diets and insulin in order to precipitate a diabetic crisis requiring hospitalization in an outside facility. This led to more guards, more expense, and more escape attempts.

A Stillwater surgeon performed common surgeries such as appendectomies, hernia repairs, and minor orthopedic procedures at the prison, and a small infirmary took care of inmates needing nursing care after surgery or for minor illnesses. Much of the nursing care was provided by inmates. I had found the Thursday-afternoon trip to the prison a change of pace from my fellowship days at the large teaching hospitals in the Twin Cities. I enjoyed the short drive in the country to meet the inmate patients.

I called the prison doctor and said, "I'll do it, but I want to see all the diabetics who take insulin and all the inmates who have complained of chest pain in the last year."

I had full clinic schedules each Thursday for several months. The general practitioner and I devised a plan to treat chest pain and out-of-control diabetics at the prison. I met with several inmates who could perform laboratory testing and act as nurses. We talked about their willingness to get up at night to evaluate inmate complaints and to run lab tests and electrocardiograms (EKGs).

Could we manage these problems safely and competently without transferring them to another facility? How would the prison population respond? Could we prevent escape attempts? It was all new ground, but we were ready to give it a try.

The first challenge came from a diabetic with high blood sugar and impending diabetic acidosis, a life-threatening state of uncontrolled diabetes. To make matters worse, he presented late in the evening when no professionally trained medical personnel were on site.

I talked to Soli, one of the inmates who worked in the prison medical lab.

"What's his blood sugar?"

"Over 300. I need to dilute it again to get a better reading."

"Any ketone bodies to indicate acidosis?"

"The stick test is positive."

We had a bad case. The inmate must have stopped his insulin shots for a day or two. Over the phone I ordered insulin, intravenous fluid and electrolytes, and a repeat blood-sugar test in one hour.

I couldn't go back to sleep, so I called the prison and reached Soli, who said,

"I'm diluting the second specimen again. The blood sugar is over 300. The stick test is still positive for ketones."

"How are his vital signs?"

"His heart rate is down to 120, blood pressure down to 130 over 85, and his respiratory rate is down to 25 a minute."

The blood tests were no better, but his vital signs suggested some response.

"Repeat the insulin dose, keep the fluid at the same rate, repeat the blood tests in two hours, and call me."

When the phone rang again, I was in a deep sleep. It took a few seconds to realize it was Soli calling.

"The blood sugar is now 275, heart rate is 100, blood pressure 100 over 60, breathing is 15, and he is sleeping."

"Keep the IV at the same rate and repeat the blood tests at 7:00 a.m. Use the sliding scale of insulin we set up last month. Give the results to the prison doctor who will be there about 8:00 a.m."

The patient recovered and was back in his cell in a few days and taking his usual dose of insulin and eating his usual diet. The prison physician managed the follow-up, and I saw the patient in my usual Thursday-afternoon clinic. We had passed the first test.

As I mentioned, I had examined most of the inmates who had heart disease or complained of chest pain. The prison physician and I developed a plan to obtain serial EKGs and blood tests for cardiac-muscle injury on any inmate presenting with chest pain that suggested a possible heart attack. We had baseline EKGs on all inmates with previous chest-pain complaints. We were ready and waiting.

Not much went unnoticed in the close confines of the prison. I got reports suggesting the five diabetics in the prison population were talking among themselves, and I expected another attempt. But it was an inmate complaining of chest pain who became the next challenge.

Late one evening, the prison physician called to say an inmate had complained of severe chest pain and shortness of breath. The initial EKG was unchanged from the baseline on record, and Soli was running blood-enzyme tests.

"Have Soli repeat the EKG in an hour and call me when he has the blood results."

When he called, the blood tests and vital signs were well within the normal limits. I asked him about the EKG.

"You know I am not trained to read EKGs. I have them laid out in front of me."

"Is the rhythm regular?"

"Yes, and the rate remains at 80 per minute."

"Any change in the V2 or V3 leads?"

"None that I can see."

"OK, continue to take vital signs every hour and repeat the EKG and blood tests in six hours. If there is any change or if you have any questions, call me. Otherwise, have the prison doctor see him in the morning."

As suspected, the case turned out to be another false alarm, but we had taken care of him at the prison. So far, our change in operations was working.

There were a couple more incidents, all at night. None required transfer from the prison facilities. Then the challenges stopped. The word was out. A prisoner could be evaluated and treated satisfactorily in the prison infirmary. Unnecessary trips to a civilian hospital were no longer an option.

One celebrity prisoner was less compliant. He was a prominent St. Paul attorney who had hired an assassin to kill his wife. The murder in an upper-class neighborhood, the trials of the two men, their convictions, and their incarcerations were all front-page news in Minnesota for several years. The lawyer was one of the chest-pain complainers who came to my clinic soon after I started. He wanted to see a cardiologist.

Heart catheterizations and surgery for coronary-artery disease were experimental at the time. We worked out a modified stress test, which he easily passed. Slowly, he became convinced that he did not have significant heart disease, and his complaints were resolved. Years later, after serving over thirty years, he was paroled, and, as far as I know, is still living in another state. To my knowledge he never developed significant heart disease.

After I had been coming to the prison for about eighteen months, I was greeted by the prison doctor as I entered the front gate.

"The warden wants to see you as soon as you come in."

"What does he want to see me about?"

"Nobody knows, but he wants to see you before your clinic."

I headed for the warden's office, passing by the main cell block. Several prisoners greeted me with, "Hi, Doc."

A guard slid open an internal gate, and an assistant led me to the warden's office. The warden stood up behind his desk and said, "Doctor Hanson, do you have any idea what you have done?"

I was startled! What was this? "I'm sorry sir, but I am at a loss for an answer."

"You saved me $150,000 last year."

In 1973 that amount of money was significant in the prison budget. He went on to explain that the savings came from his prison-guard budget allocated to outside medical care. He was also pleased there had been no further escape attempts.

My five years of practicing at Stillwater Prison came to an end in 1976. My other medical involvements became too much to continue the weekly drive. I learned a lot about prison life, and about the men paying their debts to society for some infraction of the law. The men I treated had medical problems similar to the patients I had in private practice. They had common illnesses and wanted to get better. They differed in their social histories. Many inmates had been abused in their childhood. They came from poorer neighborhoods, had less educational achievement, more dysfunctional families, and they had made poor choices of peers. There were only five men that I would not see alone in the examining room. They were the ones who were true sociopaths with few or no controls on their behavior. Society deserved to be protected from them. Inside the confined environment of the prison, they could be controlled by guards and other inmates. But on the street they could be a real threat.

(Excerpts first published in *Minnesota Medicine*, March/April 2016, p. 20–21. Reprinted by permission.)

CHAPTER TWENTY-THREE

Clearing the Air

When I started at the St. Louis Park Medical Center in 1971 as a freshly minted internist and aspiring pulmonologist (lung specialist), I expected to spend my career seeing patients. However I was soon tapped to give cardiopulmonary-resuscitation (CPR) training to physicians, nurses, therapists, and other hospital personnel. I also taught pulmonary-rehabilitation classes at Methodist Hospital in Minneapolis and with the American Lung Association of Minnesota.

When it came time to assess my goal of becoming a good internist and pulmonologist after my first five years of practice, I considered several things. I had passed the internal-medicine boards in 1972. They were challenging and required concentrated studying. I developed blurred vision in my right eye due to macular swelling, an eye condition thought to be related to stress. The stress abated and my vision improved only to recur in the other eye while preparing for the first national pulmonary-specialty boards given in 1974. Once past these milestones, my knowledge credentials were established, and my medical group made me a partner. I was receiving positive patient feedback, which indicated that I was also learning the art of medicine. Our family was settled into a comfortable home, we had enough income to make ends meet, and I took the additional position of part-time medical director of our 65-physician multispecialty-medical-group practice.

When I considered the horizon, I was interested in medical administration. But I was less drawn to volunteer teaching CPR for heart-attack victims and rehabilitating former smokers with chronic lung disease. Why should I make a major volunteer commitment to treat diseased patients after the fact? The majority of lung diseases and much heart disease were entirely preventable by eliminating the use of tobacco products. I started thinking about getting involved in smoking prevention.

Minnesota had passed a clean-indoor-air law in 1975. As the new medical director of our multispecialty group, I started implementing the law in our buildings. You have to realize the environment at that time. We had provided ashtrays for patients and families in our waiting rooms. Doctors smoked in their offices; nurses and other staff smoked in their break rooms. Patients had to answer two questions before hospital admission: "What is your insurance?" and "Do you want a smoking or nonsmoking room?" When we added a cafeteria at the main outpatient office in St. Louis Park, patients and staff lit up during coffee and lunch breaks. We were not outliers. This was the community norm.

As we implemented the new state law by designating smoking areas and banning smoking from other areas, we ran into problems. Smokers complained that they didn't have enough room, and nonsmokers complained about smoke drifting into their areas. Allowing some employees to smoke in their offices raised questions of fairness. Staff lounges became centers of conflict. Nonsmokers wanted them smoke free. Smokers did not want to go outside. The Minnesota Clean Indoor Air Act of 1975 was raising issues that were polarizing our staff.

We had a progressive pulmonary-medicine department and discussed our options. We all agreed the right thing to do was to eliminate smoking from all of our buildings and grounds. As medical director, I needed to listen to others and then act.

In 1983 I brought the smoke-free issue to our governing body, the board of trustees. As a Minnesota for-profit professional organization, the physician board had control of the enterprise. When asked for my recommendation, I swallowed hard and recommended we make all our buildings and grounds smoke free. When asked how we could do that, I responded, "I don't know, but I'm willing to learn."

As the medical director, I had been chairing departmental quality-assurance meetings for several years. Paul Batalden and Paul O'Conner led our health-services research program and helped develop processes to address quality-of-care issues. We formed a representative work group from our 300 employees and medical staff. An anonymous all-staff survey was conducted, collated, analyzed, and shared with the entire staff. We wanted to know the experiences, attitudes, and smoking status of our staff. To my surprise we had a return rate of nearly 85 percent. The internal grapevine was off and running. The survey had become a significant intervention.

The smoke-free work group analyzed the survey data, published the information in a clinic newsletter, and recommended locating one smoking area in each office building with the intent of phasing out all smoking in our buildings and grounds over two years, beginning January 1, 1986. Hallway conversations became heated, dissenters made comments to the work group and wrote letters to the governing board. But formal and informal support was also voiced.

Concentrating smoking in one area highlighted the problem. Polluted air was eliminated in waiting rooms, break rooms, offices, and lunch rooms. Surprisingly both nonsmokers and smokers supported those moves. However, we had not anticipated the severe adverse reaction to the more concentrated smoking areas. Nonsmokers found them offensive and tried to avoid them. The smokers found them inconvenient and unpleasant as they noticed the secondhand smoke was more concentrated. Employee attitudes were changing, and support for going fully smoke free was increasing.

When January 1, 1986, rolled around, the governing board, most patients, and a large majority of our workforce were supportive of a smoke-free policy in all buildings and grounds. There were dissenters, however. We complicated the process by merging with the Nicollet Clinic, another large multispecialty group of about fifty physicians, to become the Park Nicollet Medical Center.

The Nicollet Clinic had not participated in the initial decision-making process. Their medical director liked to smoke a pipe in his office. A St. Louis Park gynecologist, one of its ten founders, had been smoking cigars in his office, hallways, and, on occasion, in exam rooms for thirty years. One established cardiologist was in the habit of leaving his office every couple hours, getting in his car, and driving around several blocks while he smoked a cigarette out of sight of patients and colleagues.

I responded to multiple written complaints from staff and a few from patients. Winter seemed to highlight some of the issues for smokers. Park Nicollet became the first medical group in the country to go smoke free in all its buildings and grounds and received a citation from Surgeon General C. Everett Koop. (See photo on page 211.)

During these years the medical community began to take interest in what we were doing. I was making presentations both within and outside of our group. Methodist Hospital was a separate entity where most of our patients were hospitalized. The leadership there was not sympathetic with our cause. I was indirectly informed to refrain from bringing smoking reform to the hospital. And for good measure, I was asked not to represent the newly merged Park Nicollet Clinic on any other organizational issues. The hospital's administration was determined not to take a leadership role in the community on smoking. All the major Twin Cities hospitals were afraid of losing patients to other hospitals.

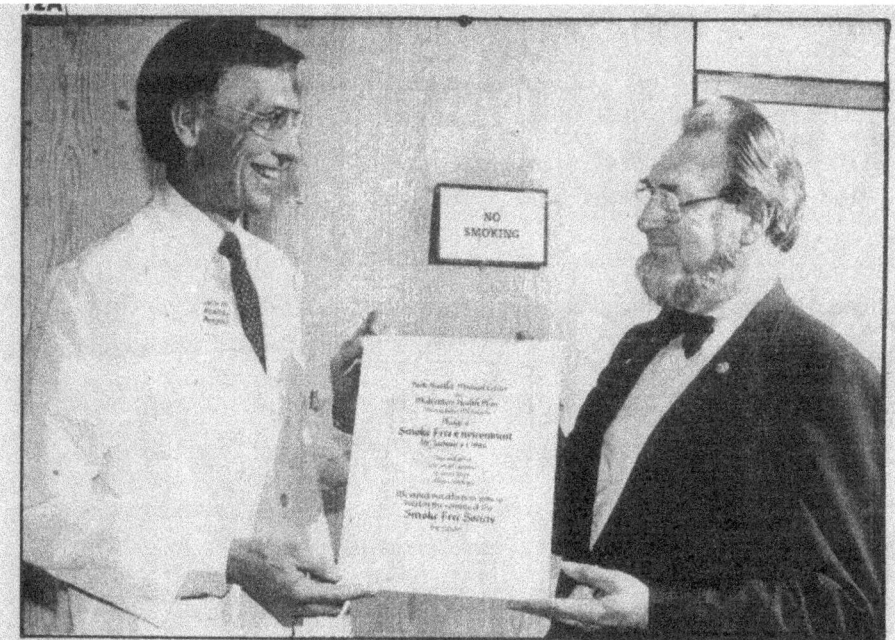

Dr. Stuart Hanson, left, presented a declaration to U.S. Surgeon General Dr. C. Everett Koop during a visit by Koop to Park Nicollet Medical Center this spring. Park Nicollet Medical Center and MedCenter Health Plans made public their plans to become smoke-free by Jan. 1, 1986 during his visit.

Reprinted with permission of Sun Sailor, *St. Louis Park, MN*

Interest in similar smoke-free initiatives was spreading and interested physicians came by to see firsthand what we were doing. In 1982 Arlene Wilson, the wife of a neurologist and a member of the Hennepin Medical Society Auxiliary, visited Norway. The Norwegian Medical Association had passed a resolution to work for a smoke-free society by the year 2000. She thought it was a good idea and asked the Hennepin County Medical Society to propose a similar resolution to the Minnesota Medical Association (MMA). When the MMA House of Delegates met in May of 1983, I was attending my first meeting as an alternate delegate to the American Medical Association (AMA) House of Delegates. Paul Blake, an independent neurosurgeon and a leader at Methodist Hospital and in the MMA, had contacted me and put my name in nomination. When I asked him why, he said, "We expect you to make a big splash."

When the Smoke-Free Society 2000 resolution passed the MMA House of Delegates that spring, an addendum was added. The Minnesota delegation was to advance this smoke-free resolution at the AMA.

The AMA House of Delegates is a large policy-making body of over 500 physicians representing state associations and specialty societies. Resolutions are debated in reference committees. Our Minnesota delegation had seven delegates and seven alternates. The chairman and several other members on the delegation were smokers. I was the new alternate attending my first meeting. When assignments were made, the chairman said, "Hanson, you're a pulmonologist. You take this damn smoking resolution."

To my surprise there were several delegates from other states who spoke in favor of our Minnesota resolution at the reference committee. The opposition seemed to come from senior physicians, some of whom were in leadership positions. By the time the resolution was on the floor, there was enough support to pass it. Now the MMA and the AMA were on record as supporting a smoke-free society by 2000. We had seventeen years to move the issue forward or to see it fade from view.

Back in Minnesota, I was asked by the MMA staff, "Now what?" My response was that we had to be credible and get our own house in order. At the time most MMA committee meetings were held at night. The meetings started with dinner and drinks from a well-supplied adult-beverage cart. Ashtrays were plentiful, and by the end of the evening, the room would be filled with smoke. Some participants would give rambling discussions and then head home, most likely in an illegal driving state. I would come home from a legislative-committee meeting to take a shower and put my smoky clothes in the washer before going to bed.

The problem was how to change this culture. I used my experience from Park Nicollet as a template, starting with a work group and a survey to assess attitudes, then designating a smoking room with the idea of going smoke free in all MMA offices and wherever MMA meetings were held. Although a few resisted, everyone knew it was the right thing to do.

Now we had some credibility to challenge other medical groups, including the AMA. Over the next two years we brought implementation resolutions and asked for progress reports. The MMA process went well and received local recognition. However, resistance was significant at the AMA. I knew that both the AMA board chair and the executive director were smokers. But when I found out that the AMA president was a closet smoker, and that the House of Delegates speaker and another board member jointly owned tobacco farms in Georgia, I knew we had taken on a major project.

C. Everett Koop, MD, was the U.S. Surgeon General at the time and had a seat in the House of Delegates. He used his position as Surgeon General as his "Bully Pulpit." When he challenged the American Lung Association at its annual meeting in April of 1984 to work for a smoke-free society by 2000, the AMA climate began to change. However, major pockets of resistance remained, which scuttled several of our efforts.

Finally, I publicly exposed the leadership's resistance and their tobacco associations at a reference-committee meeting. *The Chicago Sun-Times* newspaper picked up the story and filled in the details, including the names of the resisting leaders. The chair of the reference committee invited me to meet with the committee, and we drew up a multipoint resolution that included making the AMA offices and meetings smoke free, a position of national advocacy to support clean-air environments, and AMA promotion of smoking cessation and reduced-tobacco consumption, with an emphasis on measures to prevent youth from using tobacco products.

At this time there was a tobacco caucus and many strong anti-tobacco advocates were among the delegates. The comprehensive resolution passed and became the official policy of the AMA. The resisting leaders and delegates had lost, but did not go away immediately. At the AMA House Delegates' meetings every six months, the tobacco caucus would seek updates from the AMA staff. Gradually the organization became more in line with its mission of protecting public health. The chain-smoking chair of the board and the executive director both slowly died within the next five years of smoking-related cancer and heart disease respectively. The smoking president completed his term and did not return. I do not know what happened to the tobacco farms in Georgia.

Back in Minnesota after our first smoke-free resolution passed, our efforts did not go unnoticed. The Minnesota Department of Health (MDH) formed a task force on Smoking or Health that recommended increasing cigarette taxes and using the proceeds for a school and public education program on tobacco and health. While the task force was meeting in early 1984, Gail and I planned a sabbatical leave in Asia. We were new empty nesters, and wanted to visit family and friends in South Asia, Southeast Asia, Indonesia, China, and Japan. Gail's brother, Bob Taylor and his wife, Sue, were living in Karachi. That seemed to be a good reason to renew our association with Asia. I had been practicing pulmonary medicine at Park Nicollet for thirteen years and it was a reasonable time to reassess what we were doing with our lives and how we might live our middle-age years.

I wanted to learn firsthand how developing countries in South Asia and Southeast Asia dealt with tobacco and how they compared to developed countries like Singapore, Japan, and the United States. When we lived in Japan from 1965-68, Japanese physicians' main concern was gastric cancer. The Japanese medical industry was developing fiberoptic scopes to view and biopsy the esophagus and stomach. This was before the bacteria, Heliobacter Pylori, was known to cause stomach ulcers and before myocardial infarction was a common disease in Japan. In fact, Japanese physicians came long distances to see acute heart-attack patients at the Yokosuka Naval Hospital. At the time Japanese men had a high rate of cigarette smoking, but as a population, they had been exposed only for one or two decades and had not yet developed the major medical conditions associated with tobacco use.

What I found in Asian countries was not surprising. Health ministers and interested physicians were aware of the health consequences of unregulated tobacco use, but had little power to change much. Finance ministers overpowered health ministers. A deputy health minister in Pakistan told me the tobacco tax revenue was 7 percent of the national budget. Similar numbers were given in India, Indonesia, and Japan. No one would tell me much in China. Tuberculosis was still the major public health issue for the poorer countries. The city states of Singapore and Hong Kong were the only places where tobacco control was being addressed with public policy. One hotel in Hong Kong was the first place I knew to have both smoking and nonsmoking floors.

Thinking about the variable tobacco use in Asian countries, I began to see where the U.S. had been in the past and was headed; how ceremonial use by Native Americans and hand-rolled cigar smoking had transitioned to mass-produced products that generated billions of dollars for the growers, manufacturers, sellers, and major government receipts, but also produced millions of nicotine-addicted users. The interests of commerce were killing millions of people worldwide. Changing the course we were on would be a worthwhile investment of my time and effort. Going upstream, preventing the diseases I was treating as a physician had more appeal than trying to treat and rehabilitate the patients with heart disease, lung cancer, emphysema, and chronic obstructive lung disease that I was seeing in the office. If we were successful, I might work myself out of a job.

Back from three months in Asia I resumed my medical practice and administrative roles. I reduced my activities teaching cardiac resuscitation and pulmonary rehabilitation and delved more fully into tobacco control. I was prepared and now motivated to direct my volunteer time and efforts toward tobacco policy. I had a better understanding of how tobacco was woven into public policy of developing and developed countries. Little did I know this would become an avocation that continues.

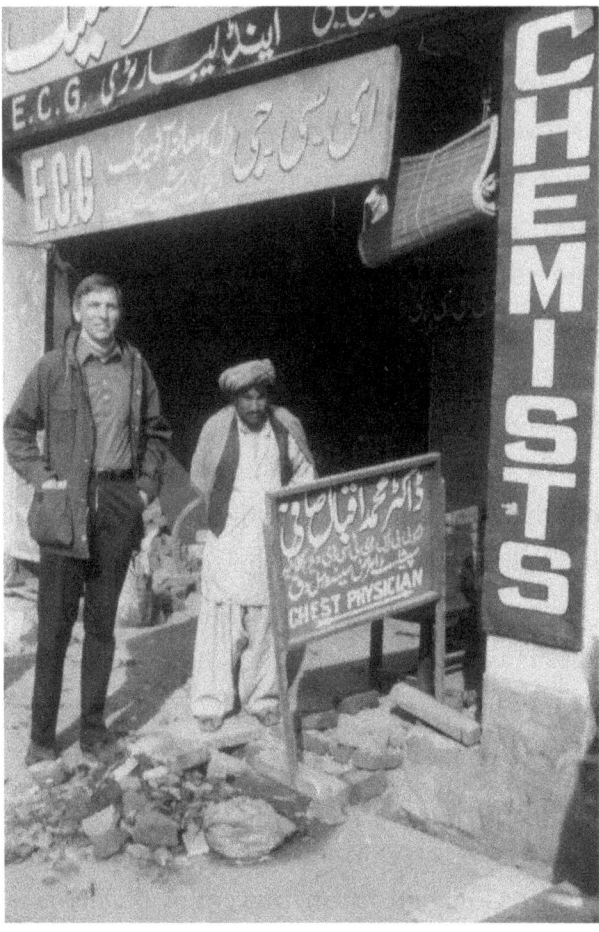

Peshawar, Pakistan, 1984, with local tobacco-activist physician at his office

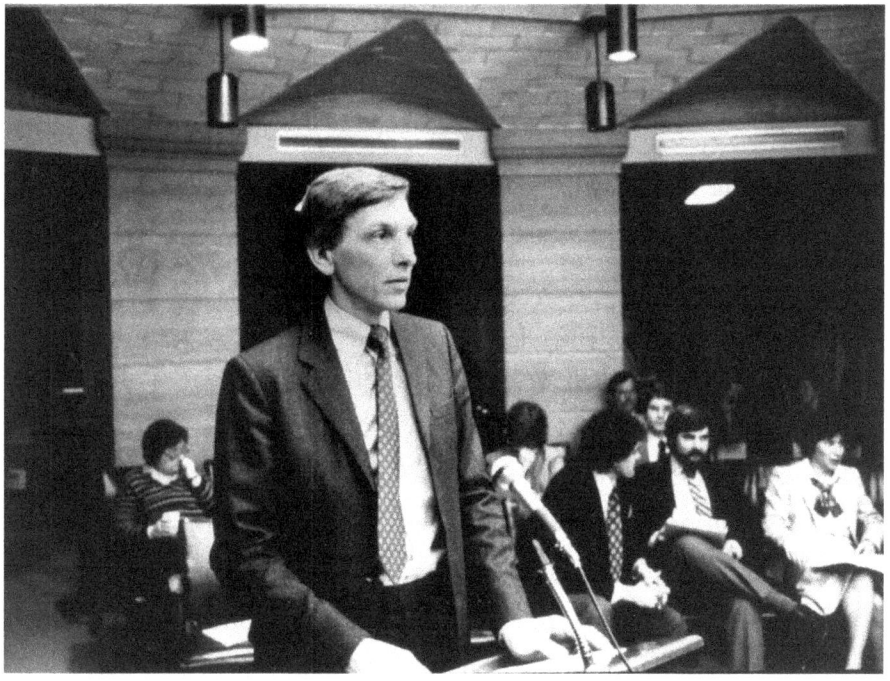

Testifying at the Minnesota State Legislature in 1985

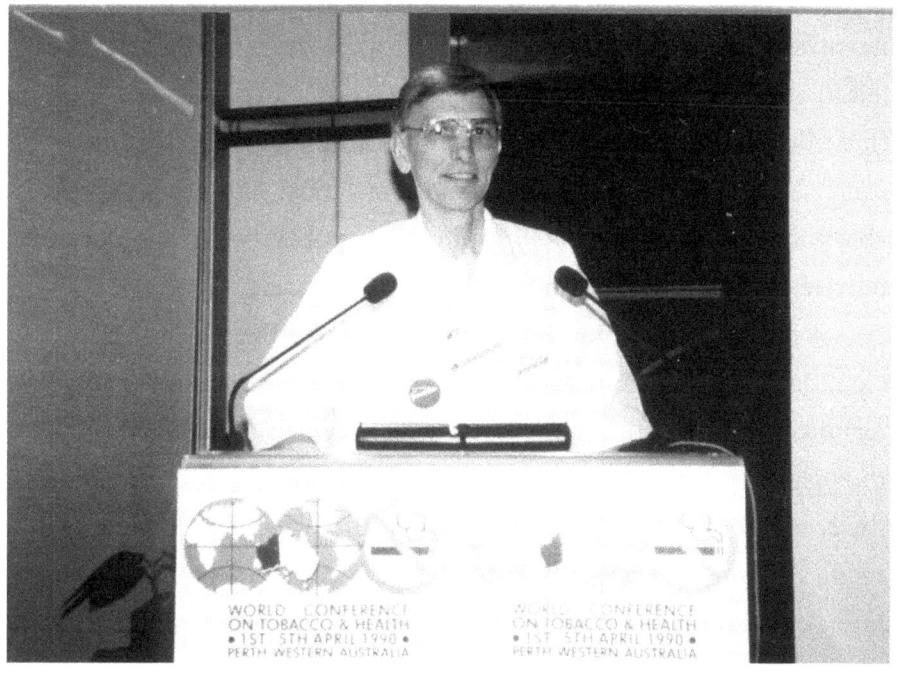

Speaking at the World Conference on Tobacco and Health, Perth, Australia, 1990

DO NO HARM

TOBACCO, HEALTH, and PUBLIC POLICY

In mid 1984 the Minnesota Department of Health Report on Smoking or Health was released. As you might expect, it was well received by the health community. Support came from the health agencies related to cancer, lung, and heart disease, the Association of Non Smokers, large medical centers like Park Nicollet and Mayo Clinics, and most of the larger Minnesota health-insurance plans.

A meeting was called by the Minnesota Department of Health (MDH). The Minnesota Medical Association (MMA), the American Cancer Society, the Minnesota Lung Association, and the Minnesota Heart Association were represented. I represented the MMA and said I thought we should address the major lifestyle behaviors including smoking, exercise, nutrition, and alcohol. We had solid evidence that changing population's approach to these lifestyle areas would have a major effect on Americans' health.

Wiser heads prevailed and the budding organization kept the focus narrowed to tobacco and smoking. The other issues would have to be left to others. (Thirty years later, we have a national obesity epidemic that Michelle Obama tried to address. Poor nutrition and lack of exercise are competing with tobacco for our most significant preventable public health problems.) In spite of my public health and political naïveté, I was selected to lead the group as president.

A nonprofit corporation, Minnesota Smoke-Free Society 2000 Coalition, was incorporated on January 1, 1985. We actually made the termination date at the end of 2000, which later had to be changed as the magic date approached. A large banquet was held to commemorate the accomplishment of getting the public and private health agencies, medical associations, health-insurance plans, and large medical groups into a cooperative effort to combat big tobacco companies in the public arena. The Surgeon General, C. Everett Koop, came to be the keynote speaker. We were off and running.

The Coalition set out a three-point mission and vision. First, all Minnesotans need to know the harmful effects of tobacco. Second, no Minnesotan should unwillingly be exposed to secondhand smoke. Third, any tobacco user should be encouraged to stop and to have access to effective support resources. This was to be a coalition of sponsoring organizations. Many were competitors for donations and prestige and had limited experience working together. The MMA gave us a desk and phone number, and a volunteer staff soon morphed into a skeleton on which to build. Managing the board was interesting and at times challenging. Those stories will not be told here.

The Minnesota legislative session in 1985 moved glacially as usual. The Department of Health had a comprehensive bill introduced. It would raise the excise tax on tobacco and dedicate the revenue to the tobacco-control initiative. When legislation gets introduced one never is sure where support or resistance may come. In this case one of the big legislative issues was how to fund state dollars to safely divert rainwater from sewer lines that emptied into the Mississippi River. Strange bedfellows, sewers and tobacco! But in retrospect they are both polluters and dangerous to health. Anyway, the health forces and the sewer forces joined to support a five-cent per pack increase in the tobacco tax. One and a half cents was dedicated to tobacco control and the rest to divert the Twin Cities' runoff water to keep the cities and towns downstream and the U.S. Federal Courts happy.

Since I was thrust into the tobacco-policy arena with the Minnesota Clean Indoor Air Act of 1975, much has changed in our state. All public buildings are now smoke free including bars and restaurants. Adult smoking rates have fallen to less than 15 percent as compared to over 30 percent in the 1970s. The state won a settlement against tobacco companies in 1997, and the proceeds are being used to fund initiatives to make quitting easier and more affordable. I became the founding president of the Minnesota Smoke Free 2000 Coalition in

1985 and in 1998 the vice chair of the Minnesota Partnership for Action Against Tobacco (now called Clearway Minnesota).

We have come a long way in the last forty years, and the work I have been involved in has been both personally and professionally satisfying. I continue to be involved in tobacco-control issues, however, the vision of a smoke-free society is still in the future. Would 2030 be a reasonable target?

(Excerpts first published in *Minnesota Medicine*, "Clearing the Air: Looking back on a public health battle." September 2015, p. 34–35. Reprinted by permission.)

CHAPTER TWENTY-FOUR

An Unexpected Reunion

Looking back to my days at Dartmouth Medical School from 1958 to 1960, I remember several stories — a first-day lecture by the dean, afternoons in the anatomy lab, attempts to keep awake during morning lectures, and our cadaver burials.

In the 1950s and 1960s Dartmouth offered the first two years of medical school. Most matriculants entered after three years of premed classes at Dartmouth College. After completing the first year of the medical school, students of the college were awarded an AB (Artium Baccalaureus) degree. After completing a second year, students received a certificate in basic medical sciences and transferred to a four-year school for the final two clinical years to earn an MD degree.

Dartmouth Medical School (currently called Geisel Medical School at Dartmouth after Theodore Geisel or Dr. Seuss) was founded in 1797, twenty-eight years after Dartmouth College. As the United States grew, medical schools proliferated. There were no national standards, no credentialing, and little accountability when medical degrees were awarded. Into this vacuum the Carnegie Foundation assigned Abraham

Flexner to make a report on medical schools in the United States and Canada. The Flexner Report of 1912 become the standard for medical education. Dartmouth Medical School soon after was judged to be deficient in clinical medical experiences and began offering only the first two basic science years. Students were required to complete the clinical years in a larger city such as Boston, New York, Baltimore, or at a home-state university.

This was the situation when twenty-three seniors in the college and one graduate came to the first-day lecture by Dean Rolf Syvertsen in September 1958. Dean Syvertsen was legendary and his first-day lectures were renowned.

"Your duty is to be here in this room at 8:00 a.m. If you're not here, the whole class will follow me down the hill to Dick's House (the college infirmary) to see you. If you're not there, we will march to the jail to bail you out, because that's where you will be. If perchance you are not there, we sadly will slowly walk to the Hanover Funeral Home to pay our respects."

Anatomy and histology were first on our agenda. We attended lectures in the morning and gross-anatomy labs in the afternoon. With some trepidation and excitement we met our cadavers the first afternoon. Twelve cadavers were laid out on separate tables. (Two other bodies were available in the morgue for future demonstrations.) The dissection room was an addition to the basement morgue and extended to the south away from the the main building. The sloping roof was made of clouded glass and reminded me of a greenhouse, except for the fact that no one could see in and nothing was growing inside. Twenty-four first-year medical students were busy dissecting out the most intimate parts of human anatomy. Two large fans placed high at the open end of the room exhausted the vapors of formaldehyde mixed with body odors of the living and the dead. As we began our first day's dissection, Charlie, the gross-anatomy and morgue attendant, sat down at the end of one of the dissection tables and ate his lunch.

AN UNEXPECTED REUNION

The 1817 education building had a main lecture hall on the first floor immediately above the morgue. In past years a false floor had allowed anatomy specimens to be lifted from the morgue to the front of the sloping classroom for demonstration. The hard seats with writing arms were probably original.

Near the building entrance a narrow, rickety stairway led to a second-floor library and museum. Long tables with old wooden chairs were surrounded by shelves and glass cases housing dusty books and large cloudy specimen jars containing human-tissue specimens long past their prime for use as teaching aids.

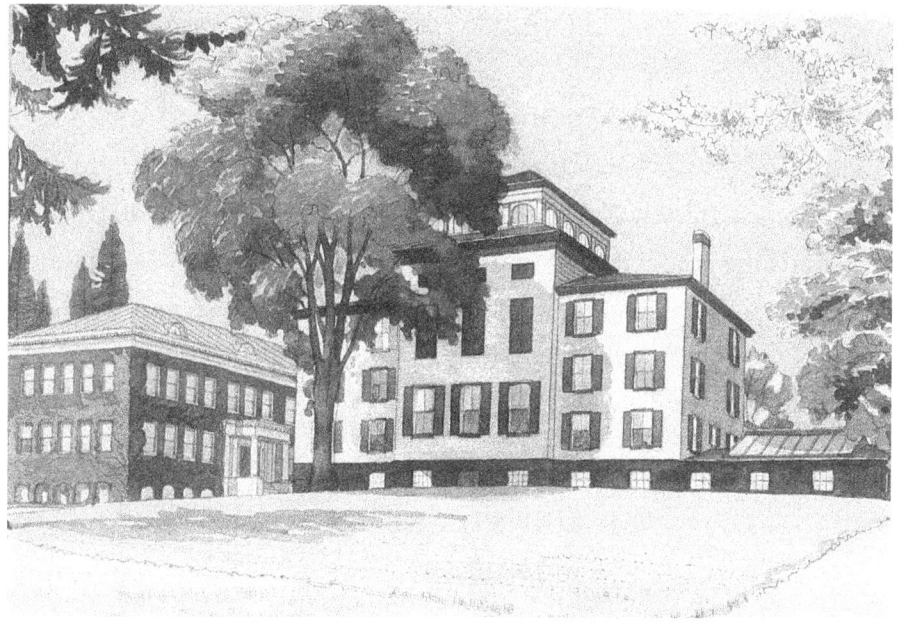

Rendering of Dartmouth Medical School as it was in the 1950s and 1960s
Courtesy of Charles Eytel, MD, Dartmouth Medical School, class of 1960
Gross-anatomy lab with glass ceiling is at the far right, histology lab was on the second floor in the building on the far left. The library museum was under the cupola in the center of the building.

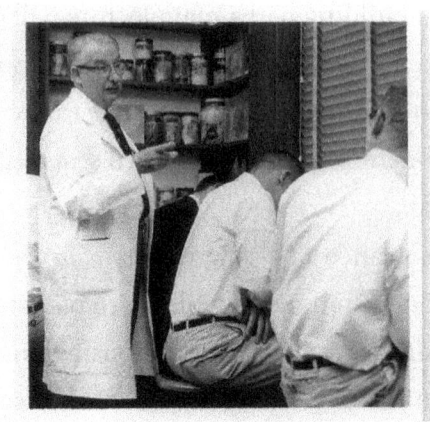

*The Dean, Dr. Rolf Syvertsen, teaching histology using monocular microscopes
Photo courtesy of Geisel Medical School at Dartmouth*

We labored into January with our scalpels, cadavers, and microscopes. Then we turned our attention to other subjects such as physiology, biochemistry, and statistics. Our relationship to our cadavers began to fade, until one day in April, at the end of class, I was handed a bulky manila envelope containing a pair of work gloves and a yellow sheet of paper with red-letter typing that read,

ANCIENT AND HONORABLE SECRET SOCIETY OF SEXTONS

ARTHUR STUART HANSON

The Ancient and Honorable Secret Society of Sextons, reposing faith in your qualifications, has unanimously elected you to membership. The enclosed secret signs are the symbols of your election.

The initiation ceremony known as the "Eight by Eight by Eight" will be holden on the afternoon and evening of Saturday, June 6, 1959.

The venerables and neophytes will assemble at the appropriate hour at the sacred vault, and will be robed in proper ceremonial garb and will carry the secret symbols.

AN UNEXPECTED REUNION

The solemn rite is one of the cardinal secrets of our Order and nothing pertaining to the ritual, time, or place may be disclosed to any non-member.

The breaking of bread will occur at the Outing Club House on Sunday, June 7, at 6:30 p.m. Attire will be informal or business suits.

Z. ERDWURM BEETLE
Grand Abbot

It took a while for me to figure out what this was all about. The gloves were the clue that we would be digging. The other "symbols" turned out to be shovels and picks. I had been "selected" as part of a team to bury our anonymous cadavers. The "Grand Abbot" was Dean Syvertsen.

On the appointed Saturday afternoon, the dean and Harry Savage, the school secretary, met us at the school and loaded eight of us, four from the second-year class of 1959, "the venerables," and four from my class of 1960, "the neophytes," into vehicles with trailers holding digging tools, "the secret symbols."

Up to this point I had no idea where we were going, but I was told the burial site was beyond the college golf course. I rode with the dean north on highway 10. Just past the golf course he turned off onto a rough, rarely used dirt trail leading to an open field overlooking the Connecticut River. Some European settlers had cleared this land for farming years before, and now it was going back to nature. There among the grasses and weeds were sets of stakes marking off eight-by-eight-foot squares designating the previous year's plots. It looked as if no one had been there since last year's sextons.

Our first task was to mark a new square just beyond last year's site. There seemed to be eight to ten plots in various stages returning to the natural state of a fallow field.

The digging of the first few feet down went fast. Gradually we began to work in shifts, careful not to throw dirt on our partners. As the hole became deeper, piles of dirt along the edge of the cavity had to be moved farther away. About six feet down, as the tallest of the "Sextons," I was elected to throw the dirt up to the edge. Now I knew why I had been selected for this task.

It was still a nice spring day when we finished digging. But, we were not through. We were to meet at the morgue at 11:00 p.m. to make the ceremonial burials at midnight. When the dean arrived, he had a larger trailer. We loaded eleven metal boxes, measuring about two-by-two-by-three feet, which contained the remains of our unidentified cadavers. The other three had been claimed by their families or friends. We knew one had been the body of a physics professor at the college.

It was a dark night and our headlights could barely find the trail to the grave site. Our crew placed the containers in the bottom of the "Eight by Eight by Eight." It was about midnight when Dean Syvertsen led a brief ceremony as we stood around our afternoon cavity that now housed steel burial containers. With the dean's "Amen," we set about using the sextons' symbols to fill the mass grave.

I remember the scene at the dinner the next evening, which didn't take place at the Outing Club House but an upper room at the College Inn. Dean Syvertsen and Harry Savage, surrounded by their student sextons, were seated at a long table, holding court. It wasn't intended to be a last supper, but sadly the dean was killed in an auto accident the following winter.

The next June, when we neophytes became venerables, we repeated the ceremony with the same symbols and a new set of neophytes. But the midnight ceremony was scrapped, and the whole event was completed in daylight. Dean Syvertsen had introduced us to the history of anatomy-specimen procurement and deposition. We didn't need to rob graves to learn human anatomy, and we really didn't need to do our burials at midnight. Or did we?

AN UNEXPECTED REUNION

Fifty-five years later, as the class of 1960 held our reunion in Hanover, much had changed. The 1817 building, where we were inducted into the medical profession, was gone. The school's name had changed, and a new hospital complex was located several miles from Hanover near the intersection of two new interstate freeways. It now is a four-year school, grants MD degrees, and has risen to prominence in many fields of medicine and health care.

Having an extra hour late one afternoon, I decided to go out to the golf course to find the field where our honored burials lie.

The golf course had some new holes on its north end. There was no dusty trail, no fallow fields of grass and weeds. I drove around trying to find something I recognized. An older, thin, grey-haired man on a bicycle had stopped near the woods to search the ground for something, perhaps mushrooms or hazelnuts.

I opened the car window, and he walked closer. "Do you know where the medical school used to bury their cadavers?" I asked.

As he moved toward my car window, he asked, "Why do you want to know?"

I explained that I had been part of a burial detail in the 1950s. His eyes lit up, and he came close. "I know where it is."

He explained in detail where to park, where to cross the fairways, and how to find the twelfth tee. "It's right behind the tee, just into the woods. Not many know it's there. The trees are the size of your leg." He gave me the directions three times, obviously wanting me to find the hidden site.

I parked my car and wove my way among the late-afternoon golfers, who may well have wondered what a lone walker was doing on their course. I stayed close to the wooded edge as I circled the eleventh green. The putters looked up as I passed. There was the twelfth tee. A foursome was ready to tee off.

They must have thought it strange to see me walking into the dense woods with neither a path (nor a golf ball) to follow.

As my eyes adjusted, I noted a broken stake among the pine and maple trees. The sun's rays came at a low angle creating shadows, making it hard to see. As I walked farther and looked back toward the tee, I made out an eight-by-eight square formed by several foot-high stakes. Then I saw a row of stakes. This was the site. The open field was being returned to the New Hampshire woods. The anonymous people buried there were going unacknowledged by the golfers passing by.

I knelt next to the first visible stake. "50," eight feet farther, "51." The metal plaques were weathered and difficult to decipher in the low light. "1957-14," "1958-11," then there it was, "1959-11." I was on my knees over eleven human remains that we young doctors-in-the-making had interred fifty-six years ago. This was a reunion I had not planned, but one full of meaning and reflection.

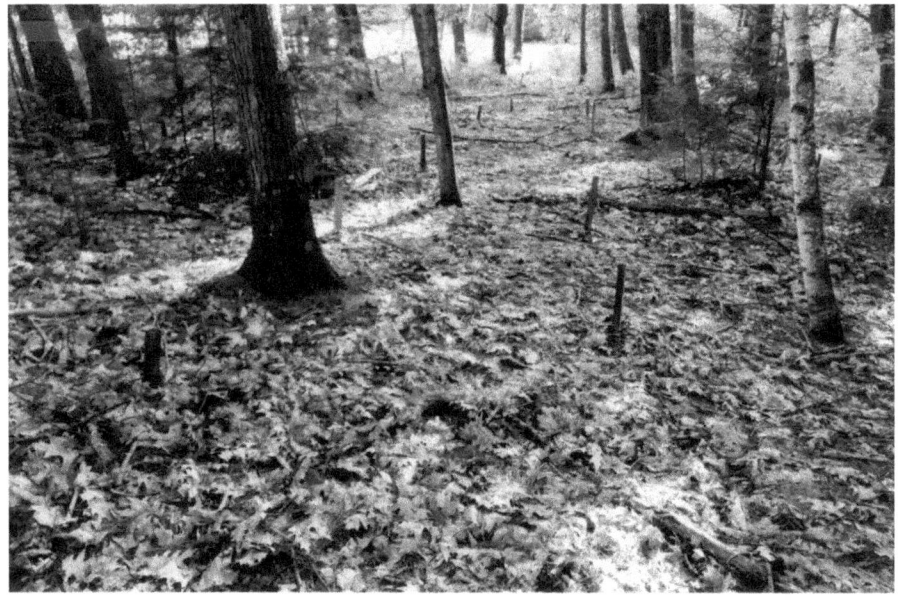

Eight-by-eight squares reaching out to a golf course beyond marking the anonymous mass graves from the 1950s and 1960s

AN UNEXPECTED REUNION

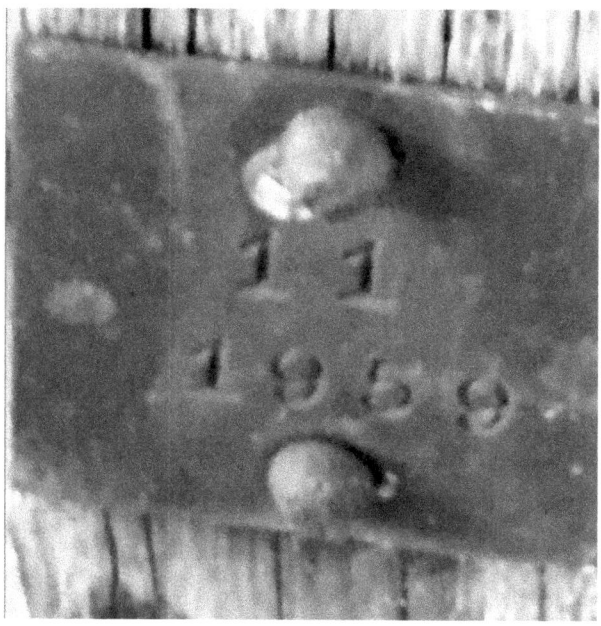

Brass plaque and stake noting the eleven individuals who contributed to the education of Dartmouth Medical School students in 1959

There were nearly 20 squares from the 1950s through the 1960s holding over 200 anonymous human remains that taught anatomy to decades of physicians. Those physicians became deans of medical schools and heads of medical departments and hospitals across the country. They researched DNA and the human genome. They surgically manipulated living human anatomies to relieve human suffering and pain. They led health-care organizations and public-health initiatives.

After this essay was initially written, the current medical school at Dartmouth cleaned out the brush at the burial grounds, trimmed the trees, and built a fence to set off the site from the golf course. A sitting bench added a place for contemplation. When they published my article in the *Geisel Medical School Alumni News*, the current practice of handling anatomic specimens was described in a sidebar. Since the 1960s, each cadaver donated to the medical school and used for research and education has been cremated and the remains either returned to the individual's family or interred in a vault at the Dartmouth Cemetery, just two miles from the burial grounds of the past. Each May, first-year medical students gather with family and friends of the deceased in the college chapel for a memorial service to remember and acknowledge the generosity of the individuals who donated their bodies to educate the next generation of physicians and to advance health care.

The reunion described here is a chapter in the human drive to understand ourselves. Medical students no longer rob graves to obtain anatomy specimens. And we no longer need to bury the remains at midnight. Our values about life and death have evolved. I think it's progress, but we cannot forget the past and the need to respect those who took part in the trajectory on which we travel.

(First published online in *Dartmouth's Geisel Medical School Alumni News*, March 2016. Reprinted by permission.)

Closing Thoughts

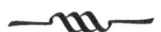

CHAPTER TWENTY-FIVE

The Final Chapter

There is one final issue to consider in the stories and thoughts that have given meaning to my life. What is the meaning of death? With my family history I could live to be one hundred. The question is what's next. I look at the answer as a journey — a spiritual journey that has taken eighty years.

I grew up in a Swedish-American family. My parents, grandparents, aunts, and uncles were all active in Swedish Lutheran churches. Sunday morning was the time for church and Sunday school. We were taught bible stories, right and wrong behavior, and could expect eternal life if we had faith in God and were good. The weekly lessons led to two years of confirmation classes and profession of faith in church doctrine and dogma as a teenager. This was not a time for deep thought about religious tenets, but a time to memorize a catechism. By the time I was in high school, I became the president of the Diamond Lake Lutheran Church youth group. I completed a Boy Scout "Pro Deo et Patria" (for God and country) service-project award by building a life-sized lighted manger scene in front of the church during a Christmas season.

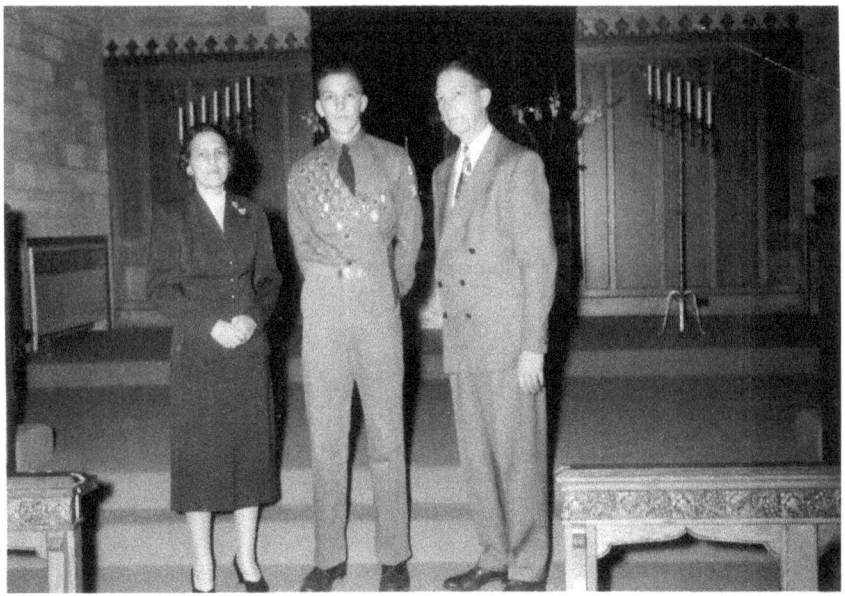

*With Mother and Dad on the day I received the
"Pro Deo et Patria" Boy Scout award*

When I started college, I joined the Lutheran Club, which was sponsored by the American Lutheran Church as a campus ministry. We met monthly on Sunday evenings in the minister's home for a home-cooked meal by his wife who was nearly our age. By my junior year, I was president of the group.

Dartmouth had several requirements the first two years. For a humanities credit, I took a course in the Judeo-Christian tradition. First we studied Catholicism, the religion of many of my boyhood friends. I found the rituals, symbols, and dogmas constraining and uninviting. I was more familiar with, and accepting of, the basic tenets of Protestantism. Then we studied Judaism, which was mostly new material for me. When the course ended, I found Judaism much more intriguing than traditional Christian religions. In the Abrahamic tradition there was one God, no Trinity, no virgin birth, and no purgatory. It was difficult to accept religious statements, creeds, and concepts of faith while I was learning the principles of science and evidence-based reasoning. I still do not understand the concept of the Holy Ghost.

THE FINAL CHAPTER

When I entered medical school at age twenty-one, I was not settled in a coherent worldview that could serve as the basis for my spiritual life. Gail and I married in the Mount Olivet Swedish Lutheran church where her mother was a member and thus we began our life together while continuing our educations and starting a family. Before we knew it, our family of four was heading off to live in Japan, while I went to sea for a year during the Vietnam War.

Going to war made me consider my place, purpose, and spiritual beliefs. What would happen if I didn't come back from one of my deployments? The first practical thing we did was to change our life insurance from an affordable savings-type policy to a term policy that provided ten times the death benefit at the same price. I was becoming more skeptical about traditional religions with confining doctrines and creeds. When Gail and I returned to Fort Snelling in the summer of 1968, I had not been formally introduced to humanism as a spiritual alternative.

I resumed my internal-medicine residency, and Gail looked for a preschool for Marta, finally settling on a Lutheran church near our apartment. Marta started to come home with the occasional proselytizing tract, and two church members came to our apartment to enlist our membership in the church. We didn't say no until they asked us to sign a creedal statement of our beliefs. We decided we could not sign something we did not believe and began to seriously consider other alternatives. Our children were growing, absorbing ideas from other adults, and we wanted them to have a welcoming place for inquiry that did not have fixed ideation. Gail's brother, Bob, and his wife, Sue, belonged to the First Universalist Church of Minneapolis, which belonged to the Unitarian Universalist Association. Unitarians had moved beyond the trinity dilemma and the Universalists found some value in all religious thought, if not their institutions. We attended a few services, enrolled Marta and Peter in Sunday school with their cousins, and became members in 1969. There were no doctrines, dogmas to accept, or pledges of faith to take. To this day the congregation recites a James Vila Blake poem to open its meetings:

> Love is the spirit of this church, and service is its law;
> this is our great covenant:
> to dwell together in peace,
> to seek the truth in love,
> and to help one another.

These simple statements, for me, embody a profound foundation for living and inquiry.

Love one another. Serve your fellow human beings and the earth, which is essential to life. Seek peace in all things. Continue learning and search for new knowledge. Serve and give back to your community. If I live by these "tenets," I feel I am a contributor not a taker, and I am living life as though I am making a difference.

How do I categorize myself after eight decades? I start by saying I am a humanist. I make decisions on rationality and scientific evidence. I do this seven days a week. I relate to others with empathy and humility. I have a responsibility to other living beings.

I have a reverence for nature. Humans are part of the natural world and its vastness and complexities are humbling and maybe beyond human comprehension. At least so far, humans have just scratched the surface of quantum mechanics (small stuff) and astrophysics (big stuff). The small and the large will continue to amaze us. I find no need to invoke a supernatural being or entity to explain our world. I call myself a "religious naturalist." At this time I have no need for a supernatural force to give me peace and comfort. That makes me a nontheist or atheist. I don't accept the idea of a controlling supernatural force, which seems to be an hypothesis without a supporting reality. Accepting a fundamental reality on the basis of faith is counter to my understanding of how the world works.

THE FINAL CHAPTER

When I retired after fifty years of learning and practicing medicine, my colleagues gave me two baseball caps. One hat said, "Every Day Is Fun," which expresses my daily optimism. When things became difficult, I would say, "Some days are more fun than others." The other hat was black with bold white lettering that read, "The End Is Near." My colleagues meant that my retirement was near. I took it to also have a second meaning about the end of life.

Most humans have contemplated the meaning of death and the possibility of an afterlife. Many institutions, mostly religious, have intellectual constructs and emotional beliefs written into their values, beliefs, and creeds. The idea of a personal afterlife is based on faith not on objective evidence. I see my afterlife embodied in the genetics I pass on, in remembrance of my actions, and in the effect I have had on other people, societal institutions, and our earth's environment. If l live this life well, that will be enough. To use a basketball metaphor, "I am in the last quarter. I have a couple of fouls, but I expect to go to the buzzer without fouling out." This will be the final chapter.

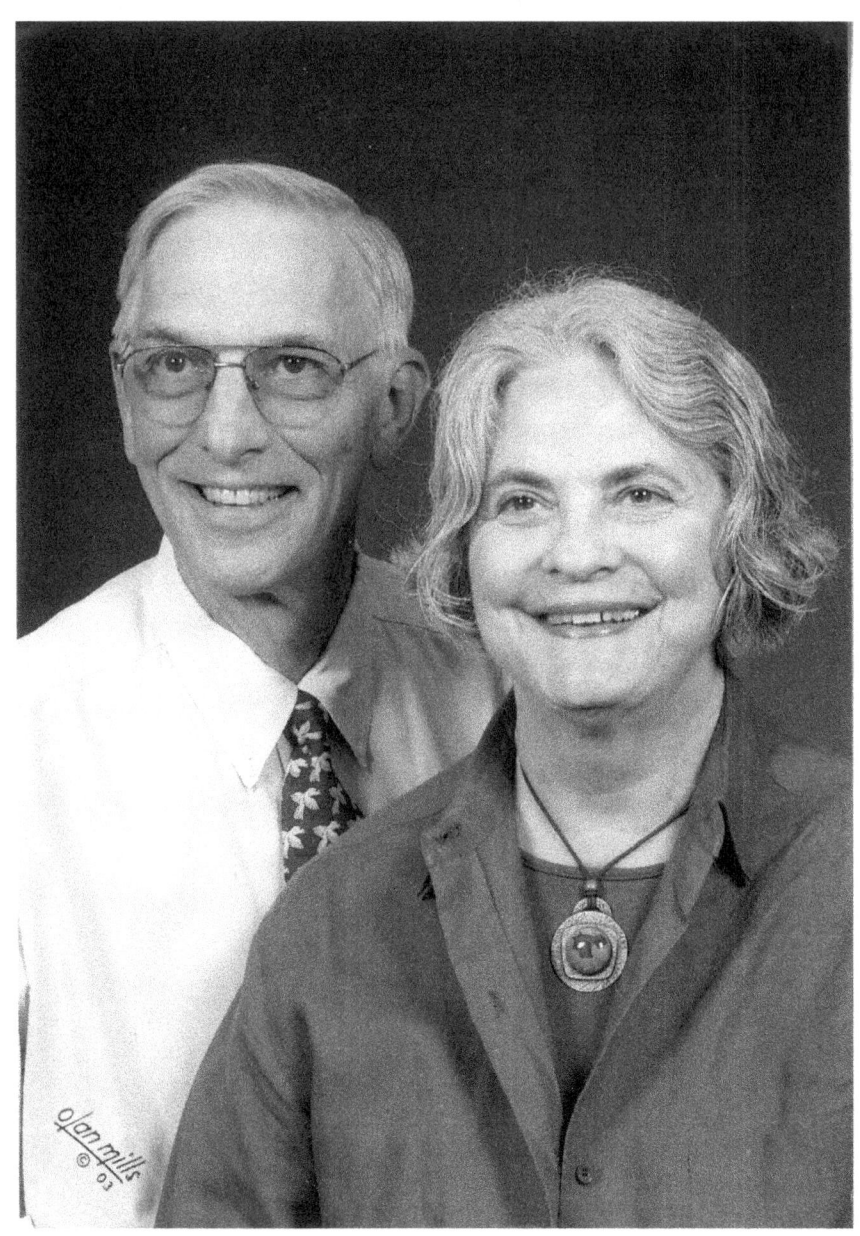

This is what the mid-seventies looked like in 2013.

CHAPTER TWENTY-SIX

Beliefs, Values, and My Lists

As the years passed, I accumulated and modified my thoughts about the world, about humanity, and about what grounded my daily activities. I tried to remember them in case anyone asked questions like, "What drives you to do what you do?" or "How do you build trust?" or "What makes a good organization?" As I got older, I had more ideas to remember. That's when I started to make lists, especially when I talked about the type of people we wanted to hire for colleagues and what kind of organizations we were trying to build. I printed these lists and kept them with my daily planner, so when I spoke, I could remember all the points.

Gradually the number of lists grew. Most of the time I didn't need them, but like an orchestra conductor or a concert musician, I had the score nearby, just in case I needed it.

When I retired as president of the Park Nicollet Institute for Research and Education in 2002, I was expected to make a speech about what I had learned about leadership and public speaking. It was not a difficult talk to give. I simply pulled out my lists and discussed the thoughts behind them. The lists represented the values I brought to work each day and how I tried to live my life day in and day out.

MY OPERATING PRINCIPLES

- You are what you do.
- Live each day as though it makes a difference.
- Live each day as though it may be your last.
- The first 100 years are the roughest.
- What you see is what you get.

BUILDING TRUST WITH OTHERS

- Make eye contact.
- Listen intently.
- Touch gently (especially patients).
- Share something about yourself.
- Laugh.
- Keep your promises.

MY CORE VALUES IN MEDICINE

- Patients come first.
- Base what you do on the best available evidence (science and reason).
- Give back to your community.

PRINCIPLES OF GOOD HEALTH

- Get upright in the morning and exercise.
- Have just enough food.
- Seek meaningful work and play.
- Maintain positive relationships with family and friends.
- Maintain enough resources. (Live below your means.)
- Sleep well and long.

ATTRIBUTES OF HEALTHY PEOPLE

- Self-respect (self-esteem) — love yourself
- Self-control (discipline)
- Respect for others — love others
- Tolerance (understanding)
- Teamwork (cooperation)
- Caring (empathy)
- Fairness (justice)
- Peaceful conflict resolution
- Social responsibility
- Generosity (altruism)

ATTRIBUTES OF HEALTHY ORGANIZATIONS

- Safe environment
- Personal respect
- Meaningful work
- Open, honest communication
- Trust (responsibility)
- Adequate resources (training)
- Constructive direction and feedback
- Recognition
- Personal growth
- Fun and enjoyment

About the Author

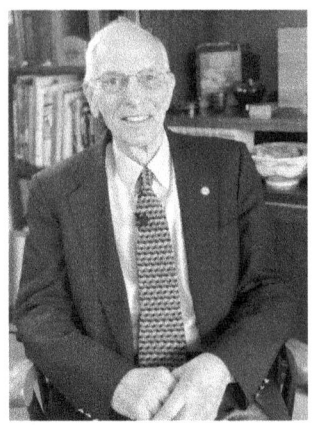

Stuart Hanson grew up in Minneapolis and attended Washburn High School. He attended Dartmouth College and completed medical school at the University of Minnesota. He served in the U.S. Navy in Vietnam and Japan. He practiced pulmonary and critical-care medicine at Park Nicollet Health Services for forty-one years before retiring in 2012. He has held leadership positions in multiple medical organizations. His public policy interests have included tobacco control, workplace behavior, health-care reform, and issues related to end-of-life care. He lives with his wife in St. Louis Park, Minnesota. They have two adult children.

www.ingramcontent.com/pod-product-compliance
Lightning Source LLC
Chambersburg PA
CBHW081937170426
43202CB00018B/2938